Surgical Practice in Rural Areas

Guest Editors

RANDALL ZUCKERMAN, MD
DAVID BORGSTROM, MD

SURGICAL CLINICS OF NORTH AMERICA

www.surgical.theclinics.com

Consulting Editor
RONALD F. MARTIN, MD

December 2009 • Volume 89 • Number 6

RS an imprint of ELSEVIER, Inc.

W.B. SAUNDERS COMPANY

A Division of Elsevier Inc.

1600 John F. Kennedy Blvd., Suite 1800, Philadelphia, PA 19103-2899

http://www.theclinics.com

SURGICAL CLINICS OF NORTH AMERICA Volume 89, Number 6

December 2009 ISSN 0039–6109, ISBN-10: 1-4377-1389-0, ISBN-13: 978-1-4377-1389-3

Editor: Catherine Bewick

Developmental Editor: Donald Mumford

Surgical Clinics of North America (ISSN 0039–6109) is published bimonthly by Elsevier Inc., 360 Park Avenue South, New York, NY 10010-1710. Months of publication are February, April, June, August, October, and December. Business and Editorial Offices: 1600 John F. Kennedy Blvd., Suite 1800, Philadelphia, PA 19103-2899. Periodicals postage paid at New York, NY and additional mailing offices. Subscription prices are $291.00 per year for US individuals, $475.00 per year for US institutions, $145.00 per year for US students and residents, $356.00 per year for Canadian individuals, $590.00 per year for Canadian institutions, $401.00 for international individuals, $590.00 per year for international institutions and $200.00 per year for Canadian and foreign students/residents. To receive student/resident rate, orders must be accompanied by name of affiliated institution, date of term, and the *signature* of program/residency coordinator on institution letterhead. Orders will be billed at individual rate until proof of status is received. Foreign air speed delivery is included in all *Clinics* subscription prices. All prices are subject to change without notice. POSTMASTER: Send address changes to *Surgical Clinics*, Elsevier Health Sciences Division, Subscription Customer Service, 3251 Riverport Lane, Maryland Heights, MO 63043. **Customer Service (orders, claims, online, change of address): Telephone: 1-800-654-2452 (U.S. and Canada); 314-447-8871 (outside U.S. and Canada). Fax: 314-447-8029. E-mail: journalscustomerservice-usa@elsevier.com (for print support); journalsonlinesupport-usa@elsevier.com (for online support).**

Reprints. For copies of 100 or more, of articles in this publication, please contact the Commercial Reprints Department, Elsevier Inc., 360 Park Avenue South, New York, New York 10010-1710. Tel. (212) 633-3812, Fax: (212) 462-1935, e-mail: reprints@elsevier.com.

The Surgical Clinics of North America is also published in Spanish by McGraw-Hill Interamericana Editores S.A., P.O. Box 5-237 06500 Mexico D.F. Mexico; and in Portuguese by Interlivros Edicoes Ltda., Rua Comandante Coelho 1085, CEP 21250, Rio de Janeiro, Brazil; and in Greek by Paschalidis Medical Publications, Athens Greece.

The Surgical Clinics of North America is covered in *MEDLINE/PubMed (Index Medicus), EMBASE/Excerpta Medica, Current Contents/Clinical Medicine, Current Contents/Life Sciences, Science Citation Index,* and *ISI/BIOMED*.

Printed in the United States of America.

Contributors

CONSULTING EDITOR

RONALD F. MARTIN, MD
Staff Surgeon, Department of Surgery, Marshfield Clinic, Marshfield, Wisconsin;
Clinical Associate Professor, University of Wisconsin School of Medicine and Public
Health, Madison, Wisconsin; Colonel, Medical Corps, United States Army Reserve

GUEST EDITORS

RANDALL ZUCKERMAN, MD, FACS
Attending Surgeon, The Hospital of Saint Raphael, New Haven, Connecticut; Consultant,
Mithoefer Center for Rural Surgery, Mithoefer Center for Rural Surgery, Cooperstown,
New York

DAVID BORGSTROM, MD, FACS
Program Director in Surgery, Mithoefer Center for Rural Surgery, Bassett Healthcare,
Cooperstown, New York

AUTHORS

DAVID. R. ANTONENKO, MD, PhD, FRCS(C), FACS
Professor of Surgery, Department of Surgery, University of North Dakota,
School of Medicine & Health Sciences, Grand Forks, North Dakota

JOSHUA D. ARNOLD, MD
Resident, Department of Surgery, University of Tennessee College of Medicine–
Chattanooga, Chattanooga, Tennessee

DAVID C. BORGSTROM, MD, FACS
Program Director in Surgery, Mithoefer Center for Rural Surgery, Bassett Healthcare,
Cooperstown, New York

TIMOTHY A. BREON, MS, MD, FACS
Chief of Staff and General Surgeon, Mahaska Health Partnership, Mahaska Health General
Surgeons, Oskaloosa, Iowa

PRESTON W. BROWN, MD, FACS
Clinical Assistant Professor, University of Tennessee College of Medicine–Chattanooga;
McMinn Surgical Group, Athens, Tennessee

MARTIN H. BRUENING, BMBS, FRACS, FRCSEd, MS
Senior Lecturer, Department of Surgery, University of Adelaide, Adelaide,
South Australia, Australia; Senior Lecturer in Surgery, Spencer Gulf Rural Health
School, University of South Australia/University of Adelaide, Whyalla Campus,
Whyalla Norrie, South Australia, Australia

R. PHILLIP BURNS, MD, FACS
Professor and Chairman, Department of Surgery, University of Tennessee College of Medicine–Chattanooga, Chattanooga, Tennessee

JOSEPH B. COFER, MD, FACS
Professor and Program Director, Department of Surgery, University of Tennessee College of Medicine–Chattanooga, Chattanooga, Tennessee

THOMAS H. COGBILL, MD, FACS
Program Director, Surgery Residency, Gundersen Lutheran Medical Foundation; Staff Surgeon, Gundersen Lutheran Health System, La Crosse, Wisconsin

KAREN DEVENEY, MD, FACS
Professor and Program Director, Department of Surgery, Oregon Health & Science University, Portland, Oregon

BRIT DOTY, MPH
Research Coordinator, Mithoefer Center for Rural Surgery, Bassett Healthcare, Cooperstown, New York

SAMUEL R.G. FINLAYSON, MD, MPH
Associate Professor of Surgery, Dartmouth Medical School, Hanover, New Hampshire; Dartmouth-Hitchcock Medical Center; The Dartmouth Institute for Health Policy and Clinical Practice, Lebanon, New Hampshire; The Mithoefer Center for Rural Surgery, Cooperstown, New York

W. HEATH GILES, MD
Resident, Department of Surgery, University of Tennessee College of Medicine–Chattanooga, Chattanooga, Tennessee

FIONA GRANT, RGN, BSc, Dip. N, MBA, MIHM
Remote and Rural Programme Manager, North of Scotland Planning Group (NoSPG), Spynie Hospital, Elgin, United Kingdom

MARK W. GUJER, MD
Chairman, Department of Anesthesia, Minnesota Institute of Minimally Invasive Surgery, Crosby, Minnesota

STEVEN J. HENEGHAN, MD
Chief of Surgery, Department of Surgery, Bassett Healthcare, Cooperstown, New York; Associate Clinical Professor, Columbia University, New York, New York

JOHN HUNTER, MD, FACS
Mackenzie Professor and Chair, Department of Surgery, Oregon Health & Science University, Portland, Oregon

ANNIE K. INGRAM, BA, LLM, PhD, FCIPD, MIHM
Project Director Remote and Rural Healthcare, United Kingdom; Director of Regional Planning & Workforce Development, NoSPG, Ashludie Hospital, Monifeith, Angus, United Kingdom

BENJAMIN T. JARMAN, MD, FACS
Associate Program Director, Surgery Residency, Gundersen Lutheran Medical
Foundation; Staff Surgeon, Gundersen Lutheran Health System, La Crosse,
Wisconsin

ERIC H. LARSON, PhD
Senior Research Scientist, MEDEX Northwest, University of Washington School
of Medicine, Seattle, Washington

THOMAS S. LAYMAN, MD, FACS
Clinical Assistant Professor, University of Tennessee College of Medicine–Chattanooga;
McMinn Surgical Group, Athens, Tennessee

TIMOTHY P. LeMIEUR, MD, FACS
Minnesota Institute for Minimally Invasive Surgery, Cuyuna Regional Medical Center,
Crosby, Minnesota

DANA CHRISTIAN LYNGE, MD
Associate Professor of Surgery, Department of Surgery, Division of General
Surgery, University of Washington School of Medicine; Research Associate,
WWAMI Rural Health Research Center, University of Washington School of Medicine,
Seattle, Washington

GUY J. MADDERN, MB, BS, FRACS, PhD, MS
R.J. Jepson Professor of Surgery, Department of Surgery, The Queen Elizabeth Hospital,
Adelaide, South Australia, Australia

HOWARD M. McCOLLISTER, MD, FACS
Co-Director, Minnesota Institute for Minimally Invasive Surgery, and Co-Director,
Bariatric Surgery Division, Minnesota Institute for Minimally Invasive Surgery,
Cuyuna Regional Medical Center, Crosby, Minnesota

DONALD E. PATHMAN, MD, MPH
Professor and Research Director, Department of Family Medicine, School
of Medicine; Director, Program on Health Professions and Primary Care,
Cecil G. Sheps Center for Health Services Research, University of North Carolina,
Chapel Hill, North Carolina

THOMAS C. RICKETTS III, PhD, MPH
Professor, Department of Health Policy and Management, School of Public Health;
Deputy Director, Cecil G. Sheps Center for Health Services Research, University
of North Carolina, Chapel Hill, North Carolina

SHAWN A. ROBERTS, MD
Minnesota Institute for Minimally Invasive Surgery, Cuyuna Regional Medical Center,
Crosby, Minnesota

PAUL A. SEVERSON, MD, FACS
Co-Director, Minnesota Institute for Minimally Invasive Surgery, and Co-Director,
Bariatric Surgery Division, Minnesota Institute for Minimally Invasive Surgery,
Cuyuna Regional Medical Center, Crosby, Minnesota

GEORGE F. SHELDON, MD
Professor of Surgery and Social Medicine, Department of Surgery, University of North Carolina; Director, American College of Surgeons Health Policy Research Institute, Chapel Hill, North Carolina

ANDREW J.W. SIM, MS, FRCS (Glasgow)
Consultant Surgeon, Western Isles Hospital, Macaulay Road, Stornoway, Isle of Lewis, Scotland, United Kingdom; Professor of Remote and Rural Medicine, University of the Highlands and Islands Millennium Institute, Ness Walk, Inverness, Scotland, United Kingdom

MICHAEL P. SUMIDA, MD, FACS
Clinical Assistant Professor, University of Tennessee College of Medicine–Chattanooga; McMinn Surgical Group, Athens, Tennessee

RANDALL ZUCKERMAN, MD
Attending Surgeon, The Hospital of Saint Raphael, New Haven, Connecticut; Consultant, Mithoefer Center for Rural Surgery, Mithoefer Center for Rural Surgery, Cooperstown, New York

Contents

> Many rural residents have limited access to surgical care. Although this problem has been ongoing for the past few decades, several factors threaten to exacerbate the situation. The narrowing of general surgery practice, workforce shortages and inappropriate distribution of surgeons, changes in how surgeons are trained, and increasing health care costs contribute to the problem. Creative approaches to address these issues are needed to provide high-quality surgical services to the approximately 50 million Americans living in rural communities.

> Almost one quarter of America's population and one third of its landmass are defined as rural and served by approximately 20% of the nation's general surgeons. General surgeons are the backbone of the rural health workforce. There is significant maldistribution of general surgeons across regions and different types of rural areas. Rural areas have markedly fewer surgeons per population than the national average. The demography of the rural general surgery workforce differs substantially from the urban general surgery workforce, raising concerns about the extent to which general surgical services can be maintained in rural areas of the United States.

> This article describes the unique roles and interrelations of general surgeons and primary care physicians in rural communities. It describes the various ways in which the work and success of the rural surgeon and the rural primary care physician rely on coordinating their efforts with the

other. It draws on available data, summary reports, and the authors' personal experiences in rural practice and fifty years of combined experience in research and policy analysis of rural health professions issues. Various issues are discussed, including the specific and unique roles that rural surgeon need to play in rural health systems, the ways in which rural surgeons relate to other physicians, and the likely consequences of not having proximal surgical services.

Physicians of all types are in short supply, with the shortage particularly acute in primary care and general surgery. As the site of the only surgery residency program in the state, Oregon Health & Science University's Department of Surgery has long been aware of the critical need for general surgeons to provide emergency and elective surgical care for those who live in remote areas and to support small rural hospitals whose survival depends on the presence of a surgeon. Based on our experience over the past 7 years, we believe that residents will benefit from a training program that provides extensive exposure to procedures unique to a rural practice. The objective of the training program is discussed in the article.

This article outlines the approach taken at Gundersen Lutheran Medical Foundation to prepare general surgery residents for rural general surgery practice. The methods focus on strong core training in general and minimally invasive surgery, additional technical skill sets, rural surgery electives, outcomes-based research experience, practice management education, and maintenance of relationships with graduates after residency.

The rural surgery rotation that is contained within the general surgery residency program at The University of Tennessee College of Medicine–Chattanooga is described in this article. The advantages of this experience, including the extensive endoscopy experience and the close exposure to practicing general surgeons, are also outlined. The rotation receives uniformly positive evaluations from residents at completion, and it has become the primary gastrointestinal endoscopy educational experience in this program. The description serves as a model that can be used by other programs to construct a rural surgery rotation.

The surgical training at Bassett is naturally broader than in many university settings, with a survey showing that nearly 70% of graduates who practice general surgery remain in a rurally designated area. Rural surgery experience falls into 3 categories: undergraduate, graduate, and postgraduate. The general surgery training program has no competing fellowships or subspecialty residencies; residents get significant experience with endoscopy; ear, nose, and throat; plastic and hand surgery; and obstetrics and gynecology. The rural setting lifestyle is valued by the students, residents, and fellows alike. It provides an ideal setting for recognizing the specific nuances of small-town American life, with a high-quality education and surgical experience.

care in rural areas. Despite these advantages, limitations that include a shortage of rural general surgeons and other surgical staff and financial constraints prevent some rural institutions from offering surgical services. Few concrete data are available on this subject, and more research is needed to confirm anecdotal reports regarding the positive economic impact derived from general surgical services. It is especially important to examine and quantify the direct and indirect financial contribution that a general surgeon makes to a rural hospital and community.

THE CLINICS ARE NOW AVAILABLE ONLINE!
Access your subscription at:
www.theclinics.com

Foreword

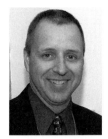

Ronald F. Martin, MD
Consulting Editor

There are many issues that contribute to the complexity of providing surgical care in a rural setting but the majority of them boil down to one common element — resource allocation or the lack thereof.

The current debate over rural surgery access and the challenges it presents is not substantially different from the larger debates over health care in general. At its core it is about how resources are allocated and who will pay for them. Smaller facilities that cannot or will not afford full-time staffing of critical needs frequently rely on their ability to transfer patients to other facilities. At what point does a medical facility's inability to staff for certain problems become the financial responsibility of another institution? How is allocating these costs decided? Should they be borne by the patient? The referring institution? The accepting institution? The municipalities involved? It is hard to say. What is clear is that at present there is a generalized expectation that transfer of a patient from one facility to another is not a financial decision although it comes with enormous financial consequences to sending and receiving facilities. Perhaps the most contentious issue we deal with in our facility, a mostly receiving facility, is providing coverage to deal with the unexpected, and the main contentious part of that issue is reimbursement.

To address this issue, first consider the barriers that are faced or imposed. Our specialty has as its primary certifier of competency the American Board of Surgery (on the allopathic side), which has struggled, largely successfully, to create a set of requirements that are highly standardized throughout North America. Our training programs are highly regulated and monitored to assure that standardized training opportunities are offered independent of the setting for training. Without doubt there is variation in training opportunities and experiences but the goal remains to homogenize the process as much as possible. Reading throughout this issue reveals that the work force requirements of practicing surgeons are markedly different from one locality to the next. Possibly the training system creates a training barrier to matching the clinical capacity to the clinical needs of some places. Specialty training addresses some of these issues for areas that can attract a large enough work force to divide responsibility but is not as effective at broadening scope of practice at present.

Surg Clin N Am 89 (2009) xiii–xiv
doi:10.1016/j.suc.2009.10.009
0039-6109/09/$ – see front matter © 2009 Elsevier Inc. All rights reserved.
surgical.theclinics.com

The ability to sort these problems is further hampered by definitions. Even the definition of rural hospital is based on the population of the town in which a hospital is located rather than its capacity. In our state, the hospital with the largest number of licensed beds is in a city with a population of only 18,000 people. Ability to stratify hospitals based on available resources, clinical service lines, and defined primary and secondary areas is not as well linked to population density as simple geographic data might imply. It seems that a series of definitions that describe hospitals based on logistic criteria might serve better.

There are some who suggest that surgeon distribution is a greater problem than surgeon shortage for covering patients in low population density areas. Whichever side of this debate one espouses does not change the fact that the basis of the delivery problem is patient access to qualified surgeons—the human capital of the system. The Balanced Budget Amendment of 1996 capped the number of (paid for) graduate medical education positions at the January 1997 level. Although there is some capacity for redistribution of specialty type within that larger total trainee number, the absolute number of general surgery residents graduated per year has remained fairly stable at slightly more than 1000. A significant fraction of these graduates pursues some form of fellowship training.

Recruitment and retention of general surgeons has become a difficult business for many areas. With a general decline in interest in frequent call obligations, increasing pressure for delivery of more types of care in "specialty centers," and a greater desire of many recent graduates to live in environments with more cultural and economic opportunities, it has become more challenging for many rural areas to compete effectively in recruiting surgeons. The obvious main incentive has been to offer greater salary subsidy but this also has its limitations.

The most likely solution, in my opinion, to the problems of "surgeon capital" allocation will be in formalizing business agreements between and among health care facilities—including their affiliated doctors. These agreements could formalize the process of transfer, provide on-site surgeon support from other institutions, or provide collaborative training efforts for maintenance of skills or maintenance of board certification. Developing these agreements may be difficult to achieve unless some external pressure forces the issue. This pressure could be mandated by government or encouraged by contractual benefit with third-party payers. As many hospitals in more rural areas provide a substantial basis for local economic activity, local businesses may generate pressure. Absent formalizing a mutually agreed-on understanding of responsibility and compensation, it seems unlikely that there will be improvement in the current dilemma.

There are many topics well covered in this issue with which we should all concern ourselves: professional isolation, differential work requirements compared to training focus, shifting desires of new surgeons for work time commitments, maintenance of critical skills, and quality control issues, to name a few. We are indebted to Dr. Zuckerman, Dr. Borgstrom, and their colleagues for assembling these articles about the problems that face rural surgeons and their patients in the United States and in other countries.

Ronald F. Martin, MD
Department of Surgery
Marshfield Clinic
1000 North Oak Avenue
Marshfield, WI 54449, USA

E-mail address:
martin.ronald@marshfieldclinic.org

Preface

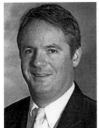 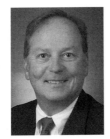

Randall Zuckerman, MD   David Borgstrom, MD
Guest Editors

The concept of "rural surgery" was a marginal issue until recently. Although sporadically discussed over the past 20 years, the problems related to the delivery of surgical services in rural areas have gained prominence in the surgical and lay literature over the past few years. This issue of *Surgical Clinics of North America* helps focus the spotlight on this important topic.

Rural surgery matters for several reasons. America and much of the world is still a predominately rural place, and the delivery of surgical care to rural residents has unique benefits and challenges. Rural surgeons may be the last bastion of true general surgery, given the broad scope of skills required for such a practice. The challenges that rural surgeons face may be forerunners of those that will have an on impact general surgery as a whole. The continued fractionation of general surgery combined with unresolved workforce issues have many worried about the ability to provide adequate surgical care to patients. This problem already exists in many rural places in the world.

Based on the emerging importance of this topic, this issue of *Surgical Clinics of North America* brings together a diverse and expert collection of authors to discuss many aspects of rural surgery ranging from very practical matters of what works to the more academic concerns of policy, outcomes, and quality. We are also fortunate to have perspectives from outside of the United States represented.

We would like to sincerely thank the contributors featured in this issue for their hard work and diligence. We would like to thank Dr Ronald Martin for the opportunity to create this issue. We would also like to thank Ms Catherine Bewick and the staff at Elsevier for their tireless work. We are also fortunate to have the support of the Mithoefer Center for Rural Surgery, which has been a beacon for research and advocacy of

Surg Clin N Am 89 (2009) xv–xvi
doi:10.1016/j.suc.2009.10.008
0039-6109/09/$ – see front matter © 2009 Elsevier Inc. All rights reserved.

surgical.theclinics.com

rural surgery. Lastly, we hope that our efforts have a positive impact on the health and surgical outcomes of rural patients.

Randall Zuckerman, MD
The Hospital of Saint Raphael
New Haven, CT 06511, USA

David Borgstrom, MD
Mithoefer Center for Rural Surgery
Bassett Healthcare
Cooperstown, NY 13326, USA

E-mail addresses:
rzuckerman@srhs.org (R. Zuckerman)
david.borgstrom@bassett.org (D. Borgstrom)

Introduction

Drs Randall Zuckerman and David Borgstrom have edited a monograph focusing on the problems and promise of rural health. A substantial portion of this evaluation deals with work force and services available. In the past, many, if not most, studies evaluated various ratios of physicians to population. Although predictions are useful to a point, each physician or health provider brings different skills to the discharge of professional services.

Predictions for the future are suspect in a rapidly changing environment. Peter Drucker, economic futurist, labeled the late twentieth and early twenty-first centuries a time of "epochal transformation." He defined epochal transformation as a period when a child would not understand the environment in which his parents lived or in which he was born. An example of a period of epochal transformation is the thirteenth century, when European society seemingly moved into cities overnight and created the bourgeoisie. In the fifteenth century, Gutenberg's invention of movable type established the printing press, and the Protestant Reformation occurred. The period of the Enlightenment in the eighteenth century brought forth the American Revolution and the writing of Adam Smith's *Wealth of Nations*. After Waterloo, the "isms" were born (ie, communism, capitalism, and so forth) along with the Industrial Revolution.[1]

The early twentieth century was characterized by World War II and the technology of atomic power; non-Western countries, such as Japan, followed by India and China, emerged as economic giants. This same period, the current period, has been characterized by transnational events, such as the fall of the Berlin Wall, the multinational war against Iraq, and so forth. Drucker has labeled this period the "knowledge society." The evolving knowledge society is transforming all elements of life as computers and robots do work.

In the early twentieth century, 40% of the population lived and worked on farms; today only 2% do so. Among the many challenges is to anticipate or predict the population dynamics and the future needs of different population centers at a time in which people under age 35 move every year and physicians, especially general surgeons, also move frequently. Confounding the problem is that 12 definitions of rural exist.[2] The use of the term, *rural*, may be classified by number of counties, population, square miles, and population per square mile. Four areas—urban, suburban, rural, and wilderness—usually cover most the parameters. In health care, health service shortage areas have been identified in most states. The basis for the classification, however, is often the presence or absence of a primary care provider and facilities. These classifications are not useful in many regions where transportation access by emergency vehicles is developed and arrangements for orderly triage occur.

There are 2052 rural counties in the United States, with 59 million citizens living rurally. These citizens are served by 1294 critical access hospitals, in which 365 counties have facilities with operating rooms but have no surgeons living in the county. Important questions are, "What is the surgical service provided and who is providing it?" Moreover, it seems clear that in many states, rural general surgeons or other surgical specialists are disappearing from small communities. How do these counties accommodate for the lack of an onsite surgeon? It is known from the National Trauma

Surg Clin N Am 89 (2009) xvii–xix
doi:10.1016/j.suc.2009.10.010
0039-6109/09/$ – see front matter © 2009 Elsevier Inc. All rights reserved.

surgical.theclinics.com

Data Bank that mortality and morbidity are higher for comparable injuries in areas remote from level I or level II trauma centers.[3] It is possible, and perhaps even likely, that treatment of other diseases, elective or chronic in nature, has less than optimal results. Forty-seven counties in North Carolina experienced a decline in the number of general surgeons to population between 1995 and 2005. Another four counties lost all general surgeons, and 18 counties had none.

Another issue is the economic viability of the rural community. Dr Thomas Ricketts estimated the direct economic impact of the average outpatient in a rural community in 2008 as between $350,000 and $500,000. An average surgeon with an inpatient practice in a small rural community contributes $1.54 to $2 million to the economic life of that community. Small rural hospitals cannot survive without surgical services and often the hospital is the largest employer in the community.

Moreover, with a population shift to the Southeast and Southwest, US and the rural to urban shift still occurring, a problem exists. The problem is for the 59 million people who live in rural America to have access to quality surgical care. Most people prefer that their surgery be done, to a degree feasible, at their local community hospital.

The problem is even more difficult considered in the light of a work force shortage of all health workers. Although growth in the number of physicians has occurred, it has not kept up with the growth of population. For general surgery, the number of physicians represents a static annual production of certified general surgeons. In 1981, 1047 general surgeons were certified by the American Board of Surgery. In 2008, the number was 1032. In 2006–2007, 7090 physicians were certified in internal medicine, with 1882 in subspecialties. In that same period, there were 2642 family medicine graduates with 287 choosing subspecialties. During the decades between 1980 and 2008, population growth was approximately 25 million each decade. For surgery, the estimated ratio in 1974 was 6.93 per 100,000 and by 2008 was probably closer to 5 per 100,000. The American Medical Association Physician Masterfile reveals a 26% drop in the general surgery work force since 1981. Of equal importance is distribution. Thompson and colleagues,[4] using the Physician Masterfile to characterize the general surgery work force in rural America, calculated the urban general surgery work force to have decreased since 1981–2005, from 14, 220 to 13,792, a drop of 27% if factored against population. The rural figures were 3135 to 2870, an even more severe drop.

There has been a fair amount of public and professional naïveté over the proper staffing and skill sets of physicians assuming a major responsibility for health care in a community. More important than specialty designation is the service provided. Internists and family medicine physicians provide many overlapping services but most cannot provide any surgical services. Surgical services are so specialized that different specialties of surgery provide little overlap. There exists a belief that prevention and primary care could obviate the need for many services, including surgical services. Certainly, primary care is needed, but it also needs to be viewed as a service and not a specialty. Institute of Medicine definitions are applicable: a definition of primary care was developed in 1978 when a committee of the Institute of Medicine, chaired by Dr E. Harvey, professor and chairman of the Department of Community and Family Medicine at Duke University, characterized five attributes: accessibility, comprehensiveness, coordination, continuity, and accountability.[5] It was noted that many primary care services are performed by specialists.

In 1994, the Institute of Medicine revised the definition of primary care as follows: primary care is the provision of integrated, accessible health care services by clinicians who are accountable for addressing a large majority of personal health care needs, developing a sustained partnership with patients, and practicing in the context of family and community.[5]

Perhaps the strongest health care trend of the past 50 years has been the decline of the solo general practitioner. Group practice is the current mode whether or not organized in a managed care vehicle or by a small private practice group. It is equally clear that the generalist in medicine is a summation of the input of different surgical and medical specialists and the input of family, advanced practice nurses, and nonphysician clinicians. The role of surgeons in this evolving paradigm is the unique service that a surgeon provides.

In this context, efforts have been attempted several times in the past to develop a rural medicine within general surgery residencies. It was anticipated that adding some obstetrics and gynecologic, orthopedic, and neurosurgery training to the core of general surgery would produce practitioners ideally suited for the rural community. In general, these experiments have not been successful. Moreover, research from the American College of Surgeons Institute for Health Policy Research indicates that the scope of practice of rural and urban general surgeons is fairly comparable. It would thus seem that the current training model, having some flexible dimensions, is probably adequate at this time. More important are the training programs in area health education centers that attract students wanting to train for a more rural practice. In the current health reform climate, expanding rural training programs and allowing surgeons to be added to primary care doctors and dentists for the benefits of the National Health Service Corps would be a useful policy. The health system are in evolution, particularly with the physician and nurse shortages, will predictably lead to more coalescence of groups and regionalization along the trauma center model. In this evolution will be the essential feature of maintaining the rural community and its needs. This timely monograph addresses the problems and promise of this changing environment. Many of these complex issues are being examined by the American College of Surgeons Health Policy Research Institute.

George F. Sheldon, MD
Department of Surgery
University of North Carolina
4006 Burnett-Womack, CB# 7050
Chapel Hill, NC 27599-7050, USA

E-mail address:
gsheldon@med.unc.edu

REFERENCES

1. Drucker PF. Post-capitalist society. New York: Harper Business/HarperCollins; 1993. p. 3.
2. Available at: http://www.ers.usda.gov/briefing/Rurality/UrbanInf. Accessed May 1, 2009.
3. Available at: http://www.facs.org/trauma/rttdc/rttdcinfo.html. Accessed May 1, 2009.
4. Thompson MJ, Lynge DC, Larson EH, et al. Characterizing the general surgery workforce in rural America. Arch Surg 2005;140:74–9.
5. Donaldson M, Yordy K, Vanselow N, editors. Defining primary care: an interim report. Washington, DC: National Academy Press; 1994.

Rural Surgery: Framing the Issues

Brit Doty, MPH[a], Randall Zuckerman, MD[a,b],*

KEYWORDS

- Rural surgery • Surgical workforce
- Surgical education • Surgical quality

The nostalgic impression of a "country doctor" captured in the work of artists, such as Norman Rockwell and W. Eugene Smith in the mid-twentieth century, remains in the minds of many decades later. All physicians, but especially surgeons, practicing in rural areas have long been considered jacks of all trades, capable of doing a bit of everything in order to take care of their patients. Often seen as willing to accept great personal sacrifice to serve the public good, work all hours of the day and night, and accept whatever payment patients could offer, the country doctor has been idealized in our history. This romantic view highlighted the attractive qualities of rural life while perhaps failing to recognize the challenges faced by rural patients and their doctors.

As early as the 1960s, several articles were published by surgeons expressing concern about the practice of rural surgery. These surgeons began the discussion of topics that continue to be addressed today, including distribution of surgeons in rural areas, challenges faced by surgeons in rural practice, types of cases performed by rural surgeons, and the education required to prepare surgeons for rural practice.[1,2] Later studies have gone on to investigate where rural residents obtain surgical services,[3] financial and reimbursement issues for rural surgeons and hospitals,[4] and quality of rural surgical care.[5] These subjects continue to be of concern and are still addressed in the literature, although current attention focuses on the larger public health goal of ensuring adequate access to surgical care for rural residents. The purpose of this article is to review the past and current rural surgery literature addressing workforce, practice, training, quality, economic, and community issues.

Funding for the Mithoefer Center and this project was received from the Robert Keeler Foundation.
[a] Mithoefer Center for Rural Surgery, Bassett Healthcare, One Atwell Road, Cooperstown, NY 13326, USA
[b] Department of Surgery, Hospital of Saint Raphael, 1450 Chapel Street, New Haven, CT 06511, USA
* Corresponding author. Department of Surgery, Hospital of Saint Raphael, 1450 Chapel Street, New Haven, CT 06511.
E-mail address: rzuckerman@srhs.org (R. Zuckerman).

Surg Clin N Am 89 (2009) 1279–1284
doi:10.1016/j.suc.2009.09.010
0039-6109/09/$ – see front matter © 2009 Elsevier Inc. All rights reserved.

DEFINING RURAL

One major question that must be addressed before turning to specific rural surgery issues is, "What is rural?" Not all rural areas are similar in terms of population density or proximity to urban centers. Using a standard definition for rural health research ensures accurate and flexible data analyses, which are critical for influencing public policy decision making.[6,7] Several methods have been developed and utilized for categorizing rural areas based on different geographic measurement units, such as counties, zip codes, and census tracts.[8] A census tract–based method tied to postal zip codes has been developed in a collaborative effort among the Health Resources and Service Administration's Office of Rural Health Policy, the Department of Agriculture's Economic Research Service, and the Washington, Wyoming, Alaska, Montana, Idaho Rural Health Research Center.[9] Rural-Urban Commuting Area Codes use standard Census Bureau urbanized area and urban cluster criteria combined with work commuting data to describe all US census tracts in terms of their rural and urban status. The 10 main Rural-Urban Commuting Area Codes and 23 underlying subcodes can be aggregated to describe different types of urban and rural communities, such as urban, large rural, small rural, and isolated rural focused areas.

DEMOGRAPHICS AND WORKFORCE ISSUES IN RURAL SURGERY

Surgical workforce issues are central to any discussion regarding rural surgery. Many health care workforce planners and surgical leaders have issued dire warnings over the past few years regarding a current and likely worsening overall shortage of general surgeons in the United States.[10–12] Findings from a study published in 2008 analyzing changes taking place in the general surgery workforce between 1981 and 2005 showed a 25% decrease in the overall number of general surgeons per 100,000 people in the United States.[13] The decline in the supply of general surgeons seems especially acute in urban and remote rural areas. Given that there is significant controversy regarding the number of physicians needed to provide high-quality health care, some health care researchers have raised questions as to whether or not a decrease in supply is akin to a shortage or whether or not the issue is actually one of maldistribution.[14,15]

Despite this ongoing debate, many people in rural areas have limited access to a general surgeon. The future seems uncertain as changes in the rural surgery workforce will likely be occurring in the next few years. Rural surgeons are on average older than their urban counterparts[16] and many will reach retirement age over the coming decade. Additionally, the vast majority of currently practicing rural surgeons are men, whereas half of graduating medical students are women. Given that women account for approximately 25% of surgical residents and few choose to practice in rural areas, the potential number of future rural surgeons may be further limited unless strategies to increase their presence in the rural setting are identified and implemented.

RURAL SURGERY PRACTICE

Several key themes are associated with the practice of rural surgery, including diverse case mix, professional isolation, frequent call coverage, and lifestyle concerns. Many publications dating back to the early 1970s describe the work of practicing rural surgeons, mainly focusing on the types of procedures they perform, from cardiac cases to thyroid procedures to laparoscopic hysterectomies, hernias, and cholecystectomies. One conclusion that can be drawn from these articles is that many surgeons practicing in rural areas seem to have a broader case mix than their urban or suburban counterparts.[17] Although adequately training new general surgeons to practice rurally may be challenging given time constraints during residency, some have argued that the ability to perform select obstetric, gynecologic, and vascular procedures could substantially expand the range of services rural surgeons are able to offer their patients.[18]

Professional isolation is a common and ongoing concern as many rural surgeons worry about maintaining infrequently used skills or learning new techniques.[19] Lack of access to mentoring and peer review opportunities can deter potential rural surgeons and prove even more daunting for young surgeons in the process of developing their skills. Another challenging issue for rural surgeons can be maintaining a balance between work and home life, especially for those practicing alone or in isolated rural areas where they are required to be on call frequently. Regions where rural surgeons can practice with partners, in multispecialty groups, or as hospital employees may be effective models to address some of these issues.

TRAINING THE RURAL SURGEON

Since 1992, the number of US medical students pursuing a general surgery career has declined,[20] with few graduates choosing to enter rural practice. There are likely several reasons for this trend, including a lack of interest in rural practice on the part of many medical students and limited training opportunities for those who are contemplating practicing rurally.[21,22] Exposing students to rural environments at some point during their medical training may be an effective way to increase interest in future rural practice regardless of specialty. A recent survey of practicing rural surgeons showed that 40% had rural exposure in medical school whereas just 11% had rural experience only during residency.[23]

As discussed previously, rural and urban/suburban surgeons differ in the breadth of cases they perform and the environment in which they practice. Because general surgeons practicing in a rural setting are likely to perform subspecialty procedures usually considered outside the realm of a typical general surgeon,[17,18,24] it would be useful if those training to work in the rural setting were exposed to a broad range of cases. Current trends in general surgery residency training, however, show that residents have performed fewer subspecialty procedures over the past 10 years.[25] In addition, the amount and quality of rural practice exposure that residents obtain during their training is highly variable even among those residencies that offer a rural training track or program.

Between 70% and 80% of graduating general surgery residents currently choose to pursue fellowship training.[26] Given time limitations during general surgery residency, this type of specialized training may be an effective means for training rural surgeons. A rural surgery fellowship could provide the opportunity to specialize and gain experience in desired subspecialty areas. Additionally, on-the-job training may be the most cost-effective and efficient method for preparing newly graduated general surgeons if this option is available in a particular community.

MEASURING QUALITY IN RURAL SURGERY

The current emphasis on health care quality and outcome measurement is not limited to hospitals or surgical practices located solely in urbanized areas.[27] Rural residents deserve the same high-quality surgical care as those living in urban or suburban communities. The American College of Surgeons National Surgical Quality Improvement Program allows hospitals and surgeons to track their outcomes but it may not be appropriate for hospitals in all geographic locales. This type of large program often uses case volume as a quality gauge, which may not be suitable in a rural, small-hospital setting.[28] Smaller, more isolated rural hospitals, especially those with low surgical volumes, may be excluded or unable to participate because of a lack of funding or staff to monitor the program. Implementation of these programs can also be expensive and time consuming for already stressed rural hospitals.

Travel to a distant hospital for surgical care is often difficult or unacceptable for rural patients, many of whom prefer to receive their medical care locally.[29] Sending surgical cases to referral centers can also have negative financial consequences are for rural hospitals, where a substantial amount, up to 30% to 40%, of billed charges derived from surgery.[30,31] One option for rural hospitals and surgeons is to utilize process-based outcome measurement programs instead of those that require large surgical case volumes.[19] Process-based quality improvement programs allow users to track and evaluate performance compared with established surgical procedure benchmarks independent of case volume.

IMPORTANCE OF RURAL SURGERY TO LOCAL HEALTH CARE SYSTEM AND ECONOMY

The impact of general surgeons on a local health care system reaches far beyond the operations they perform. Rural general surgeons provide vital surgical back-up for other physicians in specialty areas, such as obstetrics, critical care, and emergency services, including trauma. Many surgeons practicing in rural areas provide a substantial amount of primary care and consult with other local health care professionals on the management of complex patients. Rural surgeons typically perform more endoscopic procedures than their urban counterparts, including five times the number of colonoscopies.[17] Therefore, a general surgeon may be the only provider performing colonoscopy, an important cancer screening tool, for people living in rural areas without access to a gastroenterologist.

A general surgeon also provides great financial value to a rural hospital and community. Eighty-seven percent of New York State hospital administrators responding to a survey conducted in 2005 perceived general surgery services as critical to their hospital's financial viability.[32] Loss of a rural surgeon or the ability to provide surgical care can be costly for rural hospitals that rely on this in this service line to provide a significant percentage of overall revenue.[33] A rural hospital's reputation may be damaged if it is not able to offer surgical services and residents choose to bypass the local institution for care at more distant regional medical centers.[4] If patients end up at a referral center for surgical care, they may also receive other health care services there, resulting in even greater financial losses for the community hospital. This can have a negative impact on the local economy in several ways, from lower tax revenue to difficulty retaining or attracting professional community members.

SUMMARY

The issues surrounding delivery of rural surgical care are complex. As the body of research regarding the practice of surgery in rural areas has grown, it seems that further questions have evolved more quickly than answers to these problems. It is our hope that the enlightening articles in this volume of *Surgical Clinics of North America* will spark a continuing dialogue among surgeons and policy makers to begin effectively addressing the challenges that rural Americans face in obtaining surgical care.

REFERENCES

1. McVay CB. Surgery in the rural midwest: the need, the problem, and the opportunity. Arch Surg 1962;85:531–9.

2. Phillips RB. Analysis of a rural general surgical practice. Am J Surg 1968;115(6): 795–8.
3. Kane RL, Olsen DM, Newman J, et al. Giving and getting surgery in Utah: an urban-rural comparison. Surgery 1978;83(4):375–81.
4. Glenn J, Hicks LL, Daugird AJ, et al. Necessary conditions for supporting a general surgeon in rural areas. J Rural Health 1988;4(2):85–100.
5. Welch H, Larson EH, Hart LG, et al. Readmission after surgery in Washington State rural hospitals. Am J Public Health 1992;82(3):407–11.
6. Coburn AF, MacKinney AC, McBride TD, et al. Choosing rural definitions: implications for health policy. Rural Policy Research Institute Health Panel; 2007. Issue Brief #2. Available at: http://www.rupri.org/Forms/RuralDefinitionsBrief.pdf. Accessed May 6, 2009.
7. Ricketts TC, Johnson-Webb KD, Taylor P. Definitions of rural: a handbook for health policy makers and researchers. North Carolina Rural Health Research and Policy Analysis Center; 1998. Technical issue paper prepared for the Federal Office of Rural Health Policy. Available at: http://www.shepscenter.unc.edu/research_programs/rural_program/pubs/report/ruralit.pdf. Accessed May 6, 2009.
8. John PL, Reynnells L. What is rural? USDA National Library, Rural Information Center; 2008. Available at: http://www.nal.usda.gov/ric/ricpubs/what_is_rural.shtml. Accessed May 6, 2009.
9. WWAMI Rural Health Research Center. RUCA data: using RUCA. Available at: http://depts.washington.edu/uwruca/uses.html. Accessed May 6, 2009.
10. Cofer JB, Burns RP. The developing crisis in the national general surgery workforce. J Am Coll Surg 2008;206:790–7.
11. Sheldon GF. Surgical workforce since the 1975 study of surgical services in the United States. An update. Ann Surg 2007;246(4):541–5.
12. Sheldon GF. Workforce issues in general surgery. Am Surg 2007;73(2):100–8.
13. Lynge DC, Larson EH, Thompson MJ, et al. A longitudinal analysis of the general surgery workforce in the United States, 1981–2005. Arch Surg 2008;143(4): 345–50.
14. Goodman DC, Fischer ES. Physician workforce crisis? Wrong diagnosis, wrong prescription. N Engl J Med 2008;358(16):1658–61.
15. Goodman DC, Grumbach K. Does having more physicians lead to better health system performance? JAMA 2008;299(3):335–7.
16. Thompson M, Lynge DC, Larson EH, et al. Characterizing the general surgery workforce in rural America. Arch Surg 2005;140:75–9.
17. Ritchie W, Rhodes RS, Biester TW. Workloads and practice patterns of general surgeons in the United States, 1995–1997: a report from the American Board of Surgery. Ann Surg 1999;230(4):533–43.
18. VanBibber M, Zuckerman RS, Finlayson SR. Rural versus urban inpatient case-mix differences in the US. J Am Coll Surg 2006;203(6):812–6.
19. Finlayson SRG. Surgery in rural America. Surg Innov 2005;12(4):299–305.
20. National Resident Matching Program. Available at: http://www.nrmp.org/data/historicalreports.html#programresults. Accessed May 7, 2009.
21. Burkholder HC, Cofer JB. Rural surgery training: a survey of program directors. J Am Coll Surg 2007;204:416–21.
22. Doty B, Zuckerman R, Borgstrom D. Are general surgery programs likely to prepare future rural surgeons? J Am Coll Surg 2009;66(2):74–9.
23. Doty B. Women in rural surgery: demographics, practice characteristics, and perceptions about rural practice, submitted for publication.

24. Landercasper J, Bintz M, Cogbill TH, et al. Spectrum of general surgery in rural America. Arch Surg 1997;132(5):494–7.
25. Accreditation council for graduate medical education surgery case log data. Available at: http://www.acgme.org/residentdatacollection/documentation/statistical_reports.asp. Accessed May 8, 2009.
26. Stitzenberg KB, Sheldon GF. Progressive specialization within general surgery: adding to the complexity of workforce planning. J Am Coll Surg 2005;201(6): 925–32.
27. Institute of Medicine, Committee on the Future of Rural Health Care. Quality through collaboration: the future of rural health. Washington, DC: National Academy of Sciences; 2005.
28. Dimick JB, Welch HG, Birkmeyer JD. Surgical mortality as an indicator of hospital quality: the problem with sample size. JAMA 2004;292(7):847–51.
29. Finlayson SRG, Birkmeyer JD, Tosteson ANA, et al. Patient preferences for localization of care: implications for regionalization. Med Care 1999;37(2):204–9.
30. Doty BC, Heneghan S, Zuckerman R. Starting a general surgery program at a small rural critical access hospital: a case study from southeastern Oregon. J Rural Health 2007;23(4):306–13.
31. Williamson H, Hart G, Piani MJ, et al. Market shares for rural inpatient surgical services: where does the buck stop? J Rural Health 1994;10(2):70–9.
32. Zuckerman R, Doty B, Gold M, et al. General surgery programs in small rural New York State hospitals: a pilot survey of hospital administrators. J Rural Health 2006; 22(4):339–42.
33. Williamson H, Hart G, Piani MJ, et al. Rural hospital inpatient surgical volume: cutting edge service or operating on the margin? J Rural Health 1994;10(1): 16–25.

Workforce Issues in Rural Surgery

Dana Christian Lynge, MD[a,b,*], Eric H. Larson, PhD[c]

KEYWORDS

• Rural surgery • Rural surgeons • Surgeon demography
• Surgical workforce • Health workforce shortage

Almost one quarter of America's population and one third of its landmass are defined as rural. This population and area are served by approximately 20% of the nation's general surgeons.[1] They are the second most common type of physicians in rural areas after family practitioners. General surgeons are the backbone of the rural health workforce, providing crucial diagnostic and procedural backup for family practice physicians, trauma, and critical care expertise and help ensure the fiscal viability of small rural hospitals. Although the overall proportion of general surgeons working in rural areas is approximately proportional to the population of rural America, closer examination reveals significant maldistribution of general surgeons across regions and different types of rural areas. Many rural areas, in particular smaller and more remote locations, have markedly fewer surgeons per population than the national average. The demography of the rural general surgery workforce also differs substantially from the urban general surgery workforce, differences that raise serious concerns about the extent to which general surgical services can be maintained in rural areas of the United States.

GENERAL SURGERY MANPOWER IN RURAL AMERICA

The most recent nationwide comprehensive study of rural general surgical workforce was published by Thompson and colleagues[1] in 2005. They used the 2001 American Medical Association Physician Masterfile data set to identify general surgeons. They included only surgeons who listed their primary specialty as general surgery, abdominal surgery, trauma surgery, or critical care and were clinically active, finished with training, and aged 62 or younger (average age of retirement of the Fellows of the

[a] Department of Surgery, Division of General Surgery, University of Washington School of Medicine, 112 1660 South Columbian Way, Seattle, WA 98108, USA
[b] WWAMI Rural Health Research Center, University of Washington School of Medicine, 4311 11th Avenue NE, Seattle, WA, USA
[c] MEDEX Northwest, University of Washington School of Medicine, 4311 11th Avenue NE, Suite 200, Seattle, WA 98105, USA
* Corresponding author.
E-mail address: dlynge@u.washington.edu (D.C. Lynge).

Surg Clin N Am 89 (2009) 1285–1291
doi:10.1016/j.suc.2009.07.003
0039-6109/09/$ – see front matter. Published by Elsevier Inc.

surgical.theclinics.com

American College of Surgeons).[2] This definition replicated the one used by Jonasson and colleagues[3] in their landmark article on general surgical workforce published in 1995. To determine the rural or urban location of a surgeon's reported practice, they used the ZIP code version of the rural-urban commuting areas (RUCAs). The RUCAs were developed in collaboration between the Department of Agriculture's Economic Research Service and the Washington, Wyoming, Alaska, Montana, Idaho Rural Health Research Center at the University of Washington, supported by the federal Office of Rural Health Policy.[4] They use census tracts (to which ZIP codes are approximated) rather than counties to define rural areas based on community populations and journey to work commuting patterns. In the Thompson study, the 30 RUCA categories were collapsed into three groups: urban (metropolitan area core with a population greater than 50,000), large rural (large town core with a population between 10,000 and 50,000), and small or isolated rural (towns with populations of 2500 to 10,000 or areas without an urban core population of at least 2500). The differentiation between large rural and small or isolated rural proved to be a crucial development in characterizing the rural surgical workforce.

Thompson and colleagues reported that there were 6.4 surgeons per 100,000 population in 2001. In urban areas, there were 6.53 per 100,000 population. There was substantial variation in rural areas, with 7.71 per 100,000 population in large rural areas and 4.67 per 100,000 in small/isolated rural areas (**Table 1**). This discrepancy demonstrates the phenomenon, previously noted by rural health researchers, that large rural towns often constitute a health care sweet spot. Large rural areas have sufficient population to support a large referral base of primary care practitioners and crucial colleagues, such as radiologists and pathologists. In addition, surgical subspecialists who might compete with general surgeons for cases (such as vascular and thoracic surgeons and surgical oncologists) are generally concentrated in urban areas. These factors and lifestyle considerations (larger rural towns are more likely to have amenities, such as colleges, airports, and a wider variety of employment opportunities for a surgeon's spouse) may account for the higher surgeon-to-population ratio in large rural areas compared with small/isolated rural areas. Within the small/isolated rural areas, there is wide regional variation, with the number of general surgeons per 100,000 ranging from 8.04 in the New England Census Bureau Division to 3.04 in the West South Central Census Bureau Division (see **Table 1**). The western and central parts of the country tended to have the lowest numbers of surgeons per 100,000 in small or isolated rural areas (**Fig. 1**). These areas may be less attractive to surgeons for a variety of reasons: lack of a threshold population to support general surgeons, limited numbers of clinical facilities, geography, weather, and distance from major urban centers and hospitals.

THE DEMOGRAPHY OF RURAL GENERAL SURGEONS

Thompson and colleagues also examined the demographic characteristics of general surgeons—age, gender, country of medical school, and board certification—and assessed differences between those practicing in urban and rural areas (**Table 2**). They found that general surgeons older than 50 years of age were more likely to be located in small/isolated rural areas than urban areas (51.6% versus 42.1%, $P<.001$). They were also more likely to be located in small/isolated rural areas than large rural areas (51.6% versus 44.2%, $P<.001$). Female general surgeons were more likely to practice in urban areas (11.7%) than in large rural areas (6.1%) or small/isolated rural areas (7.3%) ($P<.001$). General surgeons who were international medical graduates were more likely to practice in small/isolated rural areas (25.2%) than in urban areas

Table 1
Ratios of general surgeons per 100,000 population in urban, large rural, and small/isolated rural areas of Census Bureau divisions in 2001

Census Bureau Division	Overall Number of General Surgeons	Total Population (1,000s)	Ratio	General Surgeons in Urban Areas	Population in Urban Areas (1000s)	Ratio	General Surgeons in Large Rural Areas	Population in Large Rural Areas (1000s)	Ratio	General Surgeons in Small or Isolated Rural Areas	Population in Small or Isolated Rural Areas (1000s)	Ratio
New England	981	13,407	7.32	801	11,184	7.16	62	755	8.22	118	1467	8.04
Middle Atlantic	2863	38,234	7.49	2525	33,135	7.62	161	1951	8.25	177	3147	5.62
East North Central	2721	44,034	6.18	2122	34,138	6.22	345	4496	7.67	254	5399	4.70
West North Central	1167	18,650	6.26	736	10,897	6.75	249	2775	8.97	182	4976	3.66
East South Central	1152	16,433	7.01	712	9081	7.84	235	2875	8.17	205	4476	4.58
South Atlantic	3283	48,684	6.74	2565	37,659	6.81	344	4183	8.22	374	6842	5.47
West South Central	1699	29,918	5.68	1334	21,846	6.11	227	3662	6.20	134	4409	3.04
Mountain	1024	16,760	6.11	752	12,193	6.17	161	2146	7.50	111	2420	4.59
Pacific	2353	43,287	5.44	2100	38,849	5.41	172	2520	6.82	81	1917	4.22
Total	17,243	269,411	6.40	13,647	208,985	6.53	1956	25,366	7.71	1636	35,058	4.67

Reprinted from Thompson M, Lynge D, Larson E, et al. Characterizing the general surgery workforce in rural America. Data from Arch Surg 2005;140:74–9.

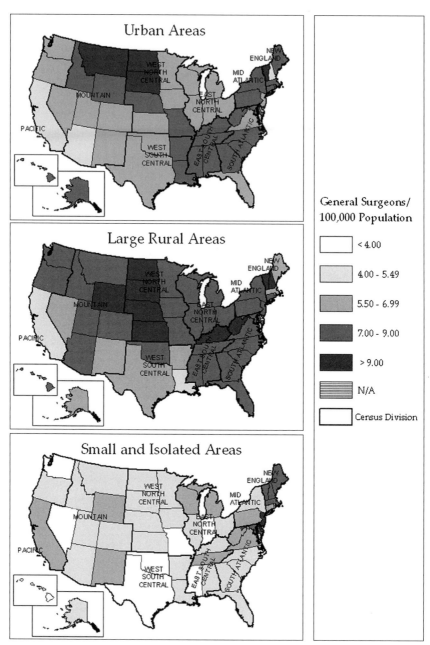

Fig. 1. General surgeon to population ratios in urban, large rural, and small/isolated areas. (*Reprinted from* Thompson M, Lynge D, Larson E, et al. Characterizing the general surgery workforce in rural America. Arch Surg 2005;140:74–9; with permission.)

Table 2
Characteristics of general surgeons in urban, large rural, and small/isolated rural areas of the United States in 2001

	Urban Areas (n = 13,647)	%	Large Rural Areas (n = 1956)	%	Small and Isolated Rural Areas (n = 1636)	%	Overall United States (n = 17,243)	%	Overall χ^2 P Value
Gender[a]									
Female	1594	11.7	120	6.1	120	7.3	1834	10.6	<0.001
Male	12,053	88.3	1836	93.9	1516	92.7	15,405	89.4	
Age (years)[a]									
<40	2753	20.2	390	19.9	249	15.2	3392	19.7	<0.001
40–49	5153	37.7	702	35.9	542	33.1	6397	37.1	
≥50	5741	42.1	864	44.2	845	51.6	7450	43.2	
Medical school[a]									
US or Canadian medical graduate	10,900	79.9	1682	86.0	1223	74.7	13,805	80.1	<0.001
International medical graduate	2747	20.1	274	14.0	413	25.2	3434	19.9	
Board certified in general surgery[b]									
Yes	10,548	94.7	1575	97.6	1180	97.7	13,303	95.2	<0.001
No	595	5.3	39	2.4	28	2.3	662	4.7	

Percentages may not add to 100 owing to rounding.
[a] Data on gender, age, and country of medical school were missing for four individuals.
[b] Data on board certification were missing for 3278 individuals.
Reprinted from Thompson M, Lynge D, Larson E, et al. Characterizing the general surgery workforce in rural America. *Data from* Arch Surg 2005;140:74–9.

(20.1%) or large rural areas (14.0%) (P<.001). The fact that general surgeons in small/isolated rural areas—many of which are already undersupplied with general surgeons compared with urban and large rural areas—are closer to retirement and less likely to be female (in an era when increasing numbers of medical students and surgeons are female) means that surgical workforce problems in these areas are likely to worsen.

TRENDS IN THE GENERAL SURGERY WORKFORCE

In a companion study to the article by Thompson and colleagues, Lynge and colleagues[5] examined trends in the general surgery workforce in the United States from 1981 to 2005. They found that the overall number of general surgeons per 100,000 population had declined by 25.91% during the past 25 years. The principal cause of the decline was the static number of general surgery residents matriculated each year for the past 2 decades despite a 1% per annum increase in population during this period.[6] Another contributing factor to the decline is the marked increase in the percentage of general surgery residents who pursue fellowship training.[7]

Small rural areas continued to have the fewest surgeons per 100,000 population and showed a steady decline of 16.31% from 1981 to 2005 (from 5.15 to 4.31 per 100,000).

In addition, the proportion of general surgeons under 40 years old declined more in rural areas than urban ones (from 25.2% to 16.8% in urban areas and from 24.5% to 13.6% in rural areas). The proportion of general surgeons aged 50 to 62 also increased more in rural areas (from 39.5% to 52%) than in urban ones (from 42.2% to 45.1%).

The proportion of general surgeons who were women increased markedly over the period of the study, from 1.4% in 1981 to 13.4% in 2005. Throughout the period covered by the study, women surgeons were more likely to be located in urban locations than rural ones. The proportion of international medical graduates decreased from 26.7% of the general surgeon population to 17.4% over the time period. In 1981, international medical graduates were almost equally distributed between urban and rural areas, but by 2005 a larger proportion were in urban areas. Large rural areas experienced the smallest rate of decline and continued to have a general surgeon–to-population ratio larger than urban or small rural places.

CURRENT AND FUTURE INFLUENCES ON SURGICAL WORKFORCE

As the older generation of general surgeons retires, it may take a larger number of surgeons to replace the more broadly trained older group.[2] The more recently trained generation of general surgeons do not typically have the training in orthopedic, obstetric, and gynecologic procedures than these retiring "omnisurgeons" do.[8,9] Another change that is already making an impact is the lack of interest of the majority of current general surgery residents in pursuing rural surgical practice, as evinced by the difficulty small rural hospitals have in recruiting general surgeons.[10] For hospitals in small and isolated rural areas of the nation—already understaffed with surgeons compared with other areas—this makes a bad situation worse. Finally, as the baby boom bulge moves into its geriatric years, an aging population will add to the workload of urban and rural surgeons.[11]

FURTHER RESEARCH ON THE RURAL SURGICAL WORKFORCE

Although the basic dimensions of the rural surgery workforce are known, important questions remain. A central problem in this field is to link provision of surgical care to surgeon density and to determine if there is a threshold rural surgeon–to-population ratio below which provision of surgical care becomes substandard. Although the health maintenance organization workforce literature[12] may provide some guidance, the nature of rural surgery and the relative lack of easy access to surgical subspecialists suggest caution in using an urban-based literature to determine the "correct" general surgeon–to-population ratio. Other important areas to examine that will affect the rural general surgical workforce and provision of surgical care include: (1) further examination of the bypass phenomenon (rural patients bypassing rural facilities and surgeons to get their surgical care at urban centers), (2) the impact of itinerant and locum tenens surgeons on the provision of surgical care in rural areas, and (3) the effect of increased penetration of surgical subspecialists into rural areas.

SUMMARY

In terms of general surgical manpower, not all rural areas are created equal. Large rural areas are well supplied compared with urban or small or isolated rural areas. Small or isolated rural areas, particularly in the western and central parts of the country, may have only two to three general surgeons per 100,000 population. Many small town and rural hospitals have no surgeon at all.

The current demography of the population of rural general surgeons does not bode well for an improvement in the workforce situation. Rural general surgeons tend to be closer to retirement than urban ones. They tend to be predominantly male in an era when more than 50% of medical students, and an increasing number of surgery residents, are female. Current general surgery graduates are increasingly choosing to subspecialize, and those who do go into general surgery tend not to go into practice in small or isolated rural areas. Rectifying this situation probably will require a complex solution that includes the following measures: (1) recruitment of medical students from rural areas who intend to go into surgery; (2) development of rural surgery training tracks with appropriate curriculums and rotations in rural locales; (3) developing debt relief incentives for newly graduated surgeons who go into rural practice; (4) eliminating any discrepancies in remuneration between urban and rural surgeons; and (5) identifying strategies that help make rural surgery a viable lifestyle choice, especially for dual-career families and female surgeons (practice-sharing options, restricted call, hospital-sponsored locums service, and so forth). These and other measures are needed to effect a fundamental shift in the way that rural surgery is practiced and makes such work more attractive to the modern surgical graduate.

REFERENCES

1. Thompson M, Lynge D, Larson E, et al. Characterizing the general surgery workforce in rural America. Arch Surg 2005;140:74–9.
2. Jonasson O, Kwakwa F, Sheldon GF. Retirement age and the workforce in general surgery. Ann Surg 1996;224:574–82.
3. Jonasson O, Kwakwa F, Sheldon GF. Calculating the workforce in general surgery. JAMA 1995;274(9):731–4.
4. Morrill R, Cromartie J, Hart L. Metropolitan, urban, and rural commuting areas: toward a better depiction of the United States' settlement system. Urban Geogr 1999;20:727–48.
5. Lynge D, Larson E, Thompson M, et al. A longitudinal analysis of the general surgery workforce in the United States, 1981–2005. Arch Surg 2008;143(4): 345–50.
6. Kwakwa F, Jonasson O. The longitudinal study of surgical residents, 1993 to 1994. J Am Coll Surg 1996;183(5):425–33.
7. Stitzenberg KB, Sheldon GF. Progressive specialization within general surgery: adding to the complexity of workforce planning. J Am Coll Surg 2005;201(6): 925–32.
8. Shively EH, Shively SA. Threats to rural surgery. Am J Surg 2005;190(2):200–5.
9. Landercasper J, Bintz M, Cogbill TH, et al. Spectrum of general surgery in rural America. Arch Surg 1997;132(5):494–6.
10. Doty B, Zuckerman R, Finlayson S, et al. How does degree of rurality impact the provision of surgical services at rural hospitals. J Rural Health 2008;24(3):306–10.
11. Etzioni DA, Liu JH, Maggard MA, et al. The aging population and its impact on the surgery workforce. Ann Surg 2003;238(2):170–7.
12. Hart L, Wagner E, Pirzada S, et al. Physician staffing ratios in staff-model HMOs: a cautionary tale. Health Aff 1997;16(1):55–70.

Interdependence of General Surgeons and Primary Care Physicians in Rural Communities

Donald E. Pathman, MD, MPH[a,c,]*, Thomas C. Ricketts III, PhD, MPH[b,c]

KEYWORDS

- Scope of practice • Preoperative care
- Postoperative management

In many rural communities, the general surgeon serves as the core—or the entirety—of the local surgical workforce.[1–4] In most rural areas, primary care physicians provide most nonsurgical medical care, including much that is provided by medical and pediatric specialists in urban areas.[5–8] Together, general surgeons and primary care physicians often play coleading roles in the health care systems of rural communities, forming the heart of the local medical workforce.[3,9]

Given their central and complementary roles, general surgeons and primary care physicians in rural communities enjoy a unique relationship.[9] Indirect evidence of their rich interactions can be found in studies and reports of surgical and trauma care in rural settings[10] and is sometimes captured in published stories about the work and lives of rural physicians.[9,11] Unfortunately, the interactions between rural surgeons and generalist physicians have not been thoroughly or systematically described[12] and they remain generally unrecognized except by those who have experienced rural health care firsthand.

This article describes the unique roles and interrelations of general surgeons and primary care physicians in rural communities. It describes the various ways in which the work and success of the rural surgeon and the rural primary care physician rely on coordinating their efforts with the other. This article draws on available data,

Funding support: none.
Potential conflicts of interest: none to report.
[a] Department of Family Medicine, School of Medicine, University of North Carolina, UNC Campus Box 7590, 725 Martin Luther King Jr, Boulevard, Chapel Hill, NC 27599-7590, USA
[b] Department of Health Policy and Management, School of Public Health, University of North Carolina, UNC Campus Box 7590, 725 Martin Luther King Jr, Boulevard, Chapel Hill, NC 27599-7590, USA
[c] Cecil G. Sheps Center for Health Services Research, University of North Carolina, UNC Campus Box 7590, 725 Martin Luther King Jr, Boulevard, Chapel Hill, NC 27599-7590, USA
* Corresponding author.
E-mail address: don_pathman@unc.edu (D.E. Pathman).

summary reports, and the authors' personal experiences in rural practice (DP) and fifty years of combined experience in research and policy analysis of rural health professions issues (DP and TR).

THE BROAD PRESENCE OF GENERAL SURGEONS AND PRIMARY CARE PHYSICIANS IN RURAL COUNTIES

General surgeons are geographically the most widely distributed of surgical specialists.[3] Indeed, there are more general surgeons per capita (7.71 per 100,000) in large rural areas than in urban areas (6.53 per 100,000).[4] Nevertheless, the distribution of general surgeons is sensitive to community size,[3] as very small communities simply cannot support a full-time surgical practice.[12,13] Hospitals in towns with fewer than 10,000 persons—the setting for most rural hospitals—have a median of only one surgeon on staff,[14] and 909 rural counties—almost one-third of all United States counties—have no surgeons at all (Ricketts TC and Belsky DW, unpublished analyses of data from the 2006 American Medical Association Masterfile and Area Resource File, US BHPr, 2007).

Physicians in primary care—family physicians, general internists, and general pediatricians—are more widely and evenly dispersed than medical and pediatric subspecialists.[3,15] Family physicians are particularly even in their distribution,[15] with 24 per 100,000 population in large urban areas, 28 per 100,000 in large rural areas, and 29 per 100,000 in rural areas with cities of less than 10,000.[3] Compared with family physicians, the per capita distribution of general internists is somewhat more sensitive to area population, with numbers of internists per 100,000 population decreasing from 42 in large urban areas, to 16 in large rural areas, and 9 in small rural areas.[3] The per capita distribution of pediatricians is even more sensitive to area population size, as their practices require a larger population base to generate adequate numbers of pediatric patients.[16,17] Pediatrician availability ranges from 21 per 100,000 population in large urban areas down to 3 per 100,000 in small rural areas.[3]

Given their ubiquitous presence in communities of all sizes, it is not surprising that family physicians form the core of the primary care physician workforce in many small rural communities.[3,15] Indeed, a 1994 study of rural hospital staffing in eight states found that among hospitals staffed by just one or two physicians, virtually all physicians were family practitioners or general practitioners.[1] Within slightly larger hospitals—those with three or four physicians on staff—general surgery was the second most commonly represented specialty, after family practice; among hospitals staffed by five or more physicians, nearly all had at least one general surgeon.

GREATER SCOPE OF PRACTICE OF SURGEONS AND PRIMARY CARE PHYSICIANS IN RURAL AREAS

Given their greater presence within rural communities and the scarcity of other physicians, general surgeons and primary care physicians often are responsible for a variety of clinical services typically provided by subspecialists within larger communities.[18,19] The urgency of some situations requires local management by whatever clinicians are available, when patients' needs for care cannot withstand a delay for transportation to reach larger medical centers and specialists.[10,20] Far more common are the many nonemergent medical situations that rural residents regard as straightforward and for which they believe that travel to distant specialists is unjustified; they simply expect local practitioners will provide this care. Time savings and convenience are valued by rural inhabitants, as for people everywhere, and some will forego needed care if not offered locally. Long travel distances and transportation difficulties are key barriers to health care access for rural inhabitants and contribute to delayed and forgone care, especially for the poor.[21]

Given the need to provide all possible and appropriate care locally, rural surgeons and primary care physicians are pushed to take on a greater scope of practice than their counterparts in urban areas.[5,9,11,12] The rural general surgeon often assumes some of the work of the gastroenterologist (eg, providing upper and lower endoscopies; managing inflammatory bowel diseases), the trauma surgeon (eg, stabilizing injuries of the chest, abdomen, and airway), the plastic surgeon (eg, repairing complex lacerations and those of sensitive neck and face structures; excising skin cancers), the orthopedic surgeon (eg, repairing flexor tendons and fractures, including some hip fractures), the pulmonologist (for bronchoscopies), and the obstetrician-gynecologist (eg, performing Cesarean sections and hysterectomies).[9,18,19,22–26] On the other hand, without the necessary specialized equipment and support staff available,[27] general surgeons in rural settings appropriately perform fewer of certain, more technical procedures than urban general surgeons, including fewer vascular procedures, pacemaker insertions, procedures of the liver and pancreas, and organ transplantations.[23,25,28]

Primary care physicians in rural settings substitute for medical specialists and other physicians and demonstrate a wider scope of practice than generalists in urban areas. The scope of practice is particularly wide for generalists in the smallest and most remote communities.[29] Compared with family physicians in urban areas, those in rural settings provide a greater proportion of their communities' care for chronic medical conditions, including heart and lung conditions, neurologic conditions, and depression.[30] They perform a wider range of diagnostic procedures such as flexible sigmoidoscopies, slit lamp evaluations, lumbar punctures, and thoracenteses; a wider variety of therapeutic procedures like endotracheal intubations, chest tube placements, vasectomies, and fracture care; and perform more women's health care procedures including obstetric deliveries, dilatation and curettage, endometrial biopsies, and intrauterine device insertions.[11,31,32] Similarly, among general internists nationwide those in smaller cities and towns more often interpret Holter monitors; manage mechanical ventilators; perform abdominal paracenteses, treadmill exercise testing, and bone barrow aspirations; and place temporary venous pacemakers.[8] The authors are unaware of data comparing the scope of practice of rural and urban pediatricians. But apart from being more often involved in children's and newborns' emergency care, the authors anticipate that the differences in scope of practice of rural and urban pediatricians are modest, since there are very few rural pediatricians in very small and remote rural communities where physicians are most pressed to broaden the services they provide, and children with less common illnesses are generally referred to urban pediatric specialists.[17,33]

THE INTERDEPENDENCE OF THE GENERAL SURGEON AND PRIMARY CARE PHYSICIAN IN RURAL COMMUNITIES

The Institute of Medicine of the National Academies and others have deemed rural settings particularly ripe for interdisciplinary collaboration.[34,35] The work of the rural surgeon uniquely compliments the work of local primary care physicians, and vice versa.[26] Consider the primary care physician staffing her or his local small hospital's emergency room (ER) on a Sunday shift. Most physician staffing of emergency departments in small hospitals is done by primary care physicians, not emergency medicine specialists.[7,36,37] The primary care physician is responsible for initiating care for all patients who present to the ER or are brought in by paramedics, including the 70-year-old man with chest pain, the infant with lethargy and dehydration, and the teenager whose flipped four-wheeler landed on his abdomen and pelvis. The physician will discharge many patients, and some she or he will admit to the small hospital to her or his own care or to the care of other local primary care physicians. Other patients, whose needs cannot be met in the small hospital, she or he will promptly stabilize and transfer to a regional referral hospital, including the elderly man with chest pain whose EKG reveals ST-segment elevation, and the injured teenager whose radiographs reveal a shattered pelvis. The physician may call in the local surgeon to assist in the evaluation, stabilization, initial care, and disposition of certain patients, including those with traumatic injuries, such as the injured teen, and those with non-traumatic surgical conditions.[9,10,26] Because there are often only one or two surgeons on staff,[14] their availability and scope of practice will factor heavily into the primary care physician's decisions regarding which patients can be appropriately managed locally and which must be transferred. If no local surgeon is available, immediate transfer becomes mandatory for all patients needing surgery, and generally appropriate for all requiring observation where surgical intervention may become necessary, including most patients with slow gastrointestinal bleeds, diverticulitis, and partial small bowel obstructions.[12] Even when a surgeon is available, his or her personal scope of practice affects whether cases that can be appropriate for some rural hospitals must be transferred from this particular hospital at this time. For example, transfer is required for a 13-year-old with appendicitis when local surgeons and anesthetists take no one under the age of 15 to the operating room, and for debridement of a soft tissue infection of the palm if the on-call local surgeon defers all hand procedures to hand specialists.[28]

Compared with urban primary care physicians, those in rural areas are generally more comfortable working without immediate specialist backup or regular medical center contact.[38,39] For many rural primary care physicians, the greater independence of rural practice is part of its appeal, allowing them to practice to the full range of their training.[11] Still, many rural generalists will be stressed by handling the multiple-trauma patient when the local general surgeon is unavailable to assist with stabilization and transfer to the regional trauma center. Anecdotally, nothing sinks the heart of the physician about to start a shift in a rural ER than spotting the sign posted above the clerk's desk that reads, "Dr Surgeon is out of town until April 30. No surgical services are available."

The availability and scope of care of the rural general surgeon are also key to the economic health of the local hospital, local primary care physicians' practices, and to the entire community.[9,12,13,40,41] A recent survey of rural hospital administrators in New York state found that 87% felt that general surgery was critical to hospital viability and 40% felt their hospitals would be forced to close if surgical services were lost.[42] Each surgical patient referred out of town is lost revenue for the local hospital and reinforces the behavior among the community's residents of bypassing the local hospital to receive care in larger, distant facilities.[12,43,44] Referring surgical patients away from the local hospital affects the practices of local primary care physicians by undermining the economic stability of their hospital and by reducing referrals for pre- and postoperative medical evaluations and management.

Within rural settings, the primary care physician is also vital to the stability of the hospital and to the work of the surgeon. The economic health of hospitals and all physicians' practices relies upon having an adequate primary care referral base for inpatient and outpatient services.[14,45] It has been estimated that a rural general surgical practice should have a referral base of at least 7 and, preferably, 11 physicians.[13]

With few medical specialists in small hospitals, rural surgeons frequently call upon primary care physicians to provide preoperative medical clearances and care, and postoperative medical management. Primary care physicians are also relied upon for in-hospital postoperative care for patients of the solo surgeon who must leave town within days of a procedure, whether for business or personal needs. The alternative for that solo surgeon is to routinely postpone all surgery for several days before leaving town, an unattractive option for both patients and surgeon. Some hospitals in communities without a surgeon arrange for itinerant surgeons to travel into town every week or two for scheduled surgeries[2,5,9,42,46,47] and then leave postoperative care to local primary care physicians.

Family physicians in many rural hospitals also assist surgeons in the operating room, filling a void created by the absence of other surgeons and midlevel providers to serve this role.[9,48] However, the proportion of United States family physicians overall—urban and rural combined—who assist in the operating room has dropped from nearly 36% in 1998[48] to 21% in 2008,[49] although the authors suspect that the fall has been less for rural family physicians.

PROFESSIONAL INTERACTIONS BETWEEN RURAL SURGEONS AND PRIMARY CARE PHYSICIANS

Compared with medical interactions within urban settings, the nature of the rural practice environment fosters closer working relationships between physicians.[35] Physicians have greater impetus to cooperate within rural settings, in part because there is often too much work to be done for everyone not to be pulling together. Rural medical communities are small and any hostilities between physicians make the inevitable interactions around patients awkward. There is simply no avoiding one another. However, with more than enough work for all physicians, there are fewer interspecialty turf battles in rural areas, allowing for more graciousness in interactions.

Rural communities' few local surgeons and primary care physicians naturally share more patients back-and-forth than is typical in urban settings, where referrals are dispersed across a wider selection of individuals practicing within a wider selection of subspecialties. Consequently, the rural surgeon and rural primary care physician communicate more regularly and depend more heavily upon one another for referrals. This makes maintaining good working relationships even more important and often yields deep and trusting partnerships, to the benefit of their practices and patient care. Within small medical communities, physicians come to learn one another's practice styles and evaluation and treatment preferences, allowing them to neatly dovetail their efforts around the evaluation, care, and referral of shared patients.

It is common for rural surgeons to teach selected surgical evaluation and technical skills to local generalists, whether around particular shared cases or through hospital-based continuing medical education programs. It is to the surgeon's advantage to ensure that primary care physicians with whom he or she works have the evaluation skills needed to prevent missed surgical diagnoses that will later complicate the work of the surgeon and to help forestall after-hours telephone consultations and referrals for minor procedures that do not require a surgeon's care. Rural surgeons also often serve leadership roles in the organization of local trauma care, emergency medical services, and training in advanced trauma life support.[10] The training they provide helps to prepare the entire health care system, including other medical staff, for the needs of the emergency and surgical patient.

Most general surgeons in rural areas augment their surgical practices by providing general medical care to patients, that is, by augmenting the primary care workforce.

Fifty-five percent of general surgeons in the rural state of West Virginia report that they provide care for the general medical problems of between 10 and 50 patients each week, including treatment of their pulmonary and cardiac diseases.[22] This practice is particularly common for surgeons in smaller West Virginia communities. Among Missouri's rural general surgeons, two-thirds report that they provide primary care services, constituting 17% of their work time, on average.[50] The proficiency of surgeons serving these roles, and the extent to which they consult their primary care colleagues or medical specialists in this work, is unknown.

PERSONAL RELATIONSHIPS BETWEEN RURAL SURGEONS AND PRIMARY CARE PHYSICIANS

With frequent referrals of patients back and forth and regular, often daily, contact, relationships between physicians can be more personal in rural settings. Physicians in rural communities can often come to know each other quite well. Professional and personal relationships blur.[51] When physicians know each other well, it becomes natural, as a matter of course, to feel and express gratitude for referrals and assistance. These relationships are a part of the close-knit nature of small towns.

In rural towns located a sizable distance away from the next nearest medical community, practitioners often serve as physicians for one another and for the care of each other's families. The primary care physician who is a professional colleague in most situations becomes the trusted personal physician for the surgeon. Conversely, the rural surgical consultant becomes the family surgeon, attending to the primary care physician's symptomatic gallstones and his or her son's inflamed appendix.

AREAS OF POTENTIAL TENSION BETWEEN RURAL SURGEONS AND PRIMARY CARE PHYSICIANS

Key in efforts to maximize the quality of surgical care for rural residents is to know which patients can be managed well within rural hospitals and which should be referred. Rural surgeons appropriately tend to refer patients needing rarely performed procedures and those needing procedures for which outcomes are more closely linked to practice volumes.[3,28] Surgical outcomes for rural hospitals have been reported to be comparable to that of urban hospitals.[10,52,53] Nevertheless, in the absence of broadly accepted, evidence-based decision rules,[54] rural primary care physicians and surgeons can sometimes differ in their opinions on which patients are appropriate for local care and which should be referred, and lower thresholds for referral have greater negative consequences for the practice of the rural surgeon. But rural primary care physicians' will also balance their referral decisions with a recognition of the importance of supporting the practice of local surgeons, whose enduring presence has broad consequences for the community's health care.

There can also be turf battles within rural communities around the overlapping content of practice of surgeons and procedurally oriented family physicians.[6,55] Generally, family physicians will fashion the scope of their services around those provided by local surgeons and other physicians. Some family physicians, for example, limit their surgical care to the field of obstetrics[46]—more often in communities where there are no obstetricians. The widest range of procedures is offered by family physicians in rural communities where there are no surgeons.[47]

While there are ample practical, interpersonal, and sociologic reasons for surgical and primary care physicians in rural communities to maintain strong and positive working relationships, the close-quartered, fishbowl environment of rural communities makes some conflict inevitable. Rural physicians are known for their independent and sometimes idiosyncratic personalities, which also makes clashes of personalities, styles, and professional judgments likely. Clashes can be found between rural physicians within and among all specialties.

THE FUTURE AND SUMMARY

The close coordination of care and frequent interactions between rural surgeons and primary care physicians stem from the unique geography and circumstances of rural communities, the limited local health care infrastructure, and few local personnel; and are influenced by situations and trends in the larger United States health care system. The relationships seen today and described in this article will change as rural and urban situations change. Evolving relationships are to be expected with the likely continued decline in numbers of general surgeons in rural communities of all sizes as more surgeons subspecialize,[15,56,57] and with the falling numbers of United States-trained family physicians and general internists.[56] Surgical and medical specialists have begun to disperse into rural counties adjacent to large urban centers,[58] which will also alter interspecialty relationships in these less remote and generally larger rural communities. Other changes in rural generalist–surgeon relationships can be expected from the ongoing expansion and reach of coordinated trauma systems and linkages to Level-III trauma centers, the decreasing numbers of family physicians trained and practicing surgical obstetrics and other major surgical procedures,[9,59] and the growth in critical-access hospitals which offer a narrower scope of services.[60] Nevertheless, it seems likely that the work of the general surgeon and primary care physician will remain particularly closely linked within the smallest and most remote rural communities into the foreseeable future. Their special relationships will likely evolve but remain uniquely rural.

With the decreasing presence of general surgeons in rural areas large and small, many rural hospitals will need to augment their surgical referral systems and arrangements with itinerant surgeons[61] or develop new ways to treat or refer these patients. This situation is, in 2009, reaching an important tipping point as there is a growing perception that there are too few physicians now being trained in many specialties and that this will affect the entire structure of health care in the United States. The specific roles of the rural surgeon and rural generalist are emblematic of the broader discussion over the appropriate balance of the physician workforce to the needs of the population and health care system.[62,63]

This article does not answer questions about which surgical services ought to be provided in rural communities or whether there are too many or too few general surgeons. Instead, this article raises various issues that can affect answers to these questions: what are the specific and unique roles that rural surgeons need to play in rural health systems, how do rural surgeons relate to other physicians, and what are the likely consequences of not having proximal surgical services? Unfortunately, too little is known about the unique roles of rural surgeons and their interactions with primary care and other physicians.[12] More information is needed on best models of care for the surgical patient in rural areas and the appropriate roles and coordination of care between rural surgeons and others.

REFERENCES

1. Krein SL, Christianson JB, Chen MM. The composition of rural hospital medical staffs: the influence of hospital neighbors. J Rural Health 1997; 13(4):306–19.

2. Larson ER, Hart LG. The rural physician. In: Geyman JP, Norris TE, Hart LG, editors. Textbook of rural medicine. New York: McGraw-Hill; 2001. p. 27–40.
3. Hart LG, Salsberg E, Phillips DM, et al. Rural health care providers in the United States. J Rural Health 2002;18(Suppl):211–32.
4. Thompson MJ, Lynge DE, Larson EH, et al. Characterizing the general surgery workforce in rural America. Arch Surg 2005;140(1):74–9.
5. Rosenblatt RA, Moscovice IS. Rural health care. New York: John Wiley & Sons; 1982.
6. Rodney WM, Hahn RG, Deutchman M. Advanced procedures in family medicine: the cutting edge or the lunatic fringe? J Fam Pract 2004;53(3):209–12.
7. McGirr J, Williams JM, Prescott JE. Physicians in rural West Virginia emergency departments: residency training and board certification status. Acad Emerg Med 1998;5:333–6.
8. Wigton RS, Nicolas JA, Blank LL. Procedural skills of the general internist. Ann Intern Med 1989;111:1023–34.
9. Lynge DC. Surgery. In: Geyman JP, Norris TE, Hart LG, editors. Textbook of rural medicine. New York: McGraw-Hill; 2001. p. 155–65.
10. Bintz M, Cogbill TH, Bacon J. Rural trauma care: role of the general surgeon. J Trauma 1996;41(3):462–4.
11. Rabinowitz HK. Caring for the country. Family doctors in small rural towns. New York: Springer; 2004.
12. Finlayson SR. Surgery in rural America. Surg Innov 2005;12(4):299–305.
13. Glenn JK, Hicks LL, Daugird AJ, et al. Necessary conditions for supporting a general surgeon in rural areas. J Rural Health 1988;4(2):85–100.
14. Doty B, Zuckerman R, Finlayson S, et al. General surgery at rural hospitals: a national survey of rural hospital administrators. Surgery 2008;143(5):599–606.
15. Council on Graduate Medical Education (COGME). Tenth report: Physician distribution and health care challenges in rural and inner-city areas. Washington, DC: Government Printing Office; 1998.
16. Committee on Careers and Opportunities. American Academy of Pediatrics. Population-to-pediatrician ratio estimates: a subject review. Pediatrics 1996;97: 597–600.
17. Randolph GD, Pathman DE. Trends in the rural-urban distribution of general pediatricians. Pediatrics 2001;107(2):e18.
18. LanderCasper J, Bintz M, Cogbill TH, et al. Spectrum of general surgery in rural America. Arch Surg 1997;132:494–7.
19. Heneghan SJ, Bordley J, Dietz PA, et al. Comparison of urban and rural general surgeons: motivations for practice location, practice patterns, and educational requirements. J Am Coll Surg 2005;201(5):732–6.
20. Rinker CF, Sabo RR. Operative management of rural trauma over a 10-year period. Am J Surg 1989;158:548–52.
21. Pathman DE, Ricketts TC, Konrad TR. How adults' access to outpatient physician services relates to the local supply of primary care physicians in the rural Southeast. Health Serv Res 2006;41:79–102.
22. Gates RL, Walker JT, Denning DA. Workforce patterns of rural surgeons in West Virginia. Am Surg 2003;69(5):367–71.
23. Ritchie WP, Rhodes RS, Biester TW. Work loads and practice patterns of general surgeons in the United States, 1995–1997: a report from the American Board of Surgery. Ann Surg 1999;230(4):533–42 [discussion: 542–3].
24. Sariego J. Patterns of surgical practice in a small rural hospital. J Am Coll Surg 1999;189(1):8–10.

25. Van Bibber M, Zuckerman R, Finlayson SRG. Rural versus urban inpatient case-mix differences in the United States. J Am Coll Surg 2005;201:S76.
26. Shively EH, Shively SA. Threats to rural surgery. Am J Surg 2005;190:200–5.
27. Cone JB. Tertiary trauma care in a rural state. Am J Surg 1990;160:652–4.
28. Dimick JB, Finlayson SR. Rural hospitals and volume standards in surgery. Surgery 2006;140(3):367–71.
29. Hutten-Czapski P, Pitblado R, Slade S. Scope of family practice in rural and urban settings. Can Fam Physician 2004;50:1548–50.
30. Moscovice KA. The practice of rural primary care. Presented at Academy Health Services Research Health Policy Meeting. Los Angeles, June 25–27, 2007.
31. Chaytors RG, Szafran O, Crutcher RA. Rural-urban and gender differences in procedures performed by family practice residency graduates. Fam Med 2001; 33(10):766–71.
32. Chen FM, Huntington J, Kim S, et al. Prepared but not practicing: declining pregnancy care among recent family medicine residency graduates. Fam Med 2006; 38(6):423–6.
33. Melzer SM, Grossman DC, Hart LG, et al. Hospital services for rural children in Washington State. Pediatrics 1997;99(2):196–203.
34. Committee on the Future of Rural Health Care. Quality through collaboration: the future of rural health care. Washington, DC: The National Academies Press; 2005.
35. Rosenthal TC, Campbell-Heider N. The rural health care team. In: Geyman JP, Norris TE, Hart LG, editors. Textbook of rural medicine. New York: McGraw-Hill; 2001. p. 41–53.
36. Peterson LE, Bazemore AW, Dodoo MS, et al. Family physicians help meet the emergency care needs of rural America. Am Fam Physician 2006;73(7):1163.
37. Moorhead JC, Gallery ME, Hirshkorn C, et al. A study of the workforce in emergency medicine: 1999. Ann Emerg Med 2002;40(1):3–15.
38. Cooper JK, Heald K, Samuels M, et al. Rural or urban practice: factors influencing the location decision of primary care physicians. Inquiry 1975;12:18–25.
39. Samaha PA, Franklin RR, Rice JC. Importance of community size in practice location decisions of final year residents. J Community Health 1987;12(2,3): 139–46.
40. Holmes GM, Slifkin RT, Randolph RK. Effect of rural hospital closures on community economic health. Health Serv Res 2006;41(2):467–85.
41. Cordes S, Van der Sluis E, Lamphear C, et al. Rural hospitals and the local economy: a needed extension and refinement of existing empirical research. J Rural Health 1999;15(2):189–201.
42. Doty B, Zuckerman R, Gold M, et al. General surgery in small rural New York hospitals. A pilot survey of hospital administrators. Available at: http://www.aamc.org/workforce/pwrc06/doty.pdf. Accessed May 6, 2009.
43. Williamson HA, Hart LG, Pirani MJ, et al. Market shares for rural inpatient surgical services: where does the buck stop? WAMI Rural Health Research Center Working Paper #21. April, 1993.
44. Liu JJ, Bellamy G, Barnet B, et al. Bypass of local primary care in rural counties: effect of patient and community characteristics. Ann Fam Med 2008;6(2):124–30.
45. Schultz DV. The importance of primary care providers in integrated systems. Healthc Financ Manage 1995;49(1):58–63.
46. Humbler N, Frecker T. Delivery models of rural surgical services in British Columbia (1996–2005): are general practitioner-surgeons still part of the picture? Can J Surg 2008;51(3):173–8.

47. Chiasson P, Roy P. The role of the general practitioner in the delivery of surgical and anesthesia services in rural western Canada. Can Med Assoc J 1995; 153(10):1447–52.
48. Hogue RL. First assisting in surgery. In: Lynge DC, Weiss BD, editors. Surgical problems and procedures in primary care. New York: McGraw-Hill Professional; 2001. p. 51–68.
49. American Academy of Family Physicians. Facts about family medicine. Available at: http://www.aafp.org/online/en/home/aboutus/specialty/facts/44.html. Accessed May 31, 2009.
50. Stevermer JJ, Supattanasiri J, Williamson H. A survey of general surgeons in rural Missouri: potential for rapid decrease in work force. J Rural Health 2001;17(1): 59–62.
51. Rich RO. The American rural metaphor: myths and realities in rural practice. Hum Serv Rural Environ 1990;14(1):31–4.
52. Galandiuk S, Mahid SS, Polk HC, et al. Differences and similarities between rural and urban operations. Surgery 2006;140(4):589–96.
53. Callaghan J. Twenty-five years of gallbladder surgery in a small rural hospital. Am J Surg 1995;169:313–5.
54. Norwood S, Fernandez L, England J. The early effects of implementing American College of Surgeons level II criteria on transfer and survival rates at a rurally based community hospital. J Trauma 1995;39(2):240–5.
55. Haynes JH, Guha SC, Taylor SG. Laparoscopic cholecystectomy in a rural family practice: the Vivian, LA, experience. J Fam Pract 2004;53(3):205–8.
56. Center for Workforce Studies. Association of American Medical Colleges. 2008 physician specialty data. Washington, DC: Association of American Medical Colleges; 2008. Available at: http://www.aamc.org/workforce/specialtyphysiciandatabook.pdf. Accessed May 31, 2009.
57. Lynge DC, Larson EH, Thompson MJ, et al. A longitudinal analysis of the general surgery workforce in the United States, 1981–2005. Arch Surg 2008;143(4): 345–50.
58. Ricketts TC, Randolph R. Urban-rural flows of physicians. J Rural Health 2007; 23(4):277–85.
59. Phillips RL, Green LA. Making choices about the scope of family practice. J Am Board Fam Pract 2002;15(3):250–4.
60. Centers for Medicaid and Medicare Services, Department of Health and Human Services. Critical Access Hospitals Center. Available at: http://www.cms.hhs.gov/center/cah.asp. Accessed May 25, 2009.
61. Doty BC, Heneghan S, Zuckerman R. Starting a general surgery program at a small rural critical access hospital: a case study from southeastern Oregon. J Rural Health 2007;23(4):306–13.
62. Cooper RA. States with more health care spending have better-quality health care: lessons about Medicare. Health Aff (Millwood) 2009;28(1):w103–15.
63. Goodman DC, Fisher ES. Physician workforce crisis? Wrong diagnosis, wrong prescription. N Engl J Med 2008;358(16):1658–61.

Education for Rural Surgical Practice: The Oregon Health & Science University Model

Karen Deveney, MD*, John Hunter, MD

KEYWORDS

- Surgical education • General surgery residency
- Rural surgery • Surgery training • Rural surgical practice

Like many states in the United States, Oregon has a large rural area with a lower physician-to-population ratio than in the urban and metropolitan central core of the state. In 2004, the Portland area had 302 physicians per 100,000 population, whereas the rural counties in the northwest part of the state had only 104 physicians per 100,000 population.[1] Physicians of all types are in short supply, with the shortage particularly acute in primary care and general surgery. As the site of the only surgery residency program in the state, Oregon Health & Science University's (OHSU's) Department of Surgery has long been aware of the critical need for general surgeons to provide emergency and elective surgical care for those who live in remote areas and to support the small rural hospitals whose survival depends on the presence of a surgeon.

Several studies have documented that the cases performed by rural general surgeons differ markedly from those that are performed in urban hospitals and that the typical urban general surgery residency does not offer trainees the breadth of cases in surgical specialties that they will need if they desire to practice in a rural, remote setting, whether domestic or international.[2–4]

NEEDS ASSESSMENT

In the mid-1990s, we realized that rural surgeons were aging and were, in many cases, unable to attract newly graduated general surgeons to join them. We conducted a needs assessment of rural hospitals and surgeons to identify how critical that need was. We found that the average age of the practicing surgeons was 47 years and that many of them were seeking surgical partners to join their practices,

Department of Surgery, Oregon Health & Science University, 3181 SW Sam Jackson Park Road, Mailcode L223, Portland, OR 97239, USA
* Corresponding author.
E-mail address: deveneyk@ohsu.edu (K. Deveney).

Surg Clin N Am 89 (2009) 1303–1308
doi:10.1016/j.suc.2009.07.007
0039-6109/09/$ – see front matter © 2009 Elsevier Inc. All rights reserved.

but they were having difficulty identifying individuals who desired or felt comfortable in a rural practice. We asked them to list the types of cases that they had performed over the past 2-year period and found that most of their practice consisted of gastro-intestinal endoscopy. In addition to the common general surgery operations, these general surgeons performed simple gynecologic, urologic, head and neck, hand, and orthopedic procedures. Most of these surgeons had not been trained to do these procedures during their residency, but, in most cases, had learned them from senior partners after entering rural practice. They felt that specific training in the procedures that are commonly performed in a rural setting and also the experience obtained in a rural setting itself would help alleviate the reluctance that general surgeons might have in entering the otherwise uncharted territory of a rural general surgery practice. Although we explored the possibility of an elective rural experience in a small community or communities, identifying the most appropriate site and securing the funding were problematic. Another issue of concern was that the site could not be too small or else it would not offer an appropriate range of surgical experience during a short rotation. We also recognized that a rotation of the usual length of 6 weeks would be too brief to provide a true sampling of life in a rural setting.

INITIAL STEPS

In 2001, the ideal solution to our problems arose when a resident from a moderate-sized rural community in Oregon suggested the possibility of spending an elective year in his hometown of Grants Pass, Oregon, which has a 125-bed hospital and 8 board-certified general surgeons and also has board-certified specialty surgeons in the fields of gynecology, otolaryngology, urology, and orthopedic surgery. Grants Pass is a town with a population of 23,000, in a forested area located 250 miles from Portland. Although it is not a remote "frontier" community, it has a definite small-town feeling and fits the Oregon definition of a rural community as one with a population of less than 30,000 located more than 50 miles from a community of more than 50,000 people. In addition, the hospital administration was supportive and was willing to fund the resident's experience. The absence of competing learners in surgical subspecialties also contributed to the resident's exposure to the basic procedures in the surgical specialties.

The first resident of the program had grown up in the community and had previously worked with some of the surgeons when he was in high school and college. He spent the academic year of 2002 to 2003 in Grants Pass in lieu of his research year, which occurs after the third clinical year of residency in OHSU's general surgery residency. The first resident's experience in Grants Pass was so positive for the resident and the community that a second fourth-year resident spent the following year there instead of his research year.

The experience of these residents included more than 50 endoscopic procedures, a broad range of general surgery operations, and direct experience with evaluation and management of emergencies in surgical specialties. The residents had rotations in obstetrics/gynecology, orthopedics, otolaryngology, and urology in which they saw patients in the office and in the emergency room. They learned (1) to manage ovarian masses, ectopic pregnancies, tubo-ovarian abscesses, and pelvic inflammatory disease; (2) to perform cesarean sections, laparoscopic tubal ligations, and oophorectomies; (3) to reduce and cast fractures, evaluate and manage hand injuries, and excise peritonsillar abscesses; (4) to manage nephrolithiasis, evaluate hematuria, and perform vasectomies and orchiectomies; and (5) to place difficult Foley catheters.

The initial 2 residents each performed 250 to 300 major operations during their practice in Grants Pass.

The experience was so successful for both the residents and for the Three Rivers Community Hospital in Grants Pass that they wished to add a second resident to the program. We also applied to the Residency Review Committee in Surgery to add Three Rivers Community Hospital as a hospital where our residents could rotate for a year as the fourth clinical year of their residency.

The educational rationale for the addition of the Three Rivers Community Hospital to our program was clear: in a state with the tenth largest land mass in the United States and a large rural area, but a small and shrinking number of rural surgeons, there was a need for well-trained surgeons in our rural communities. Also, there was an interest on the part of a small but motivated group of residents to gain skills that would allow them to practice effectively in such settings. In addition, several residents wished to spend a part of their career or their entire career in international settings, which also requires a broader depth of surgical experience than what they will learn in the typical academic general surgery program. Before they committed to a rural practice, they needed to experience what life in a rural setting would be like for them and their families. A short rotation length neither provides this experience nor does it allow the hospital staff and community to gain familiarity and trust with the individual. A 1-year experience provided the resident a greater chance to see acute problems in the surgical specialties that are important to know how to treat but that occur infrequently. A short rotation length would give little exposure to the specialties.

CURRENT EDUCATIONAL PROGRAM

Specific learning objectives of the program are listed in **Table 1**.

The resident spends 4 to 6 weeks in each of 4 formal rotations: gynecology, urology, orthopedics, and otolaryngology. They spend the remainder of the year working with the general surgeons in that community, all of whom are board-certified and are committed to working with the resident. The 2 residents alternate home call for their patients and for the emergency room. They attend office hours with their preceptors, seeing their own patients and new patients of the practice. They also learn about office management, the "business of medicine," and how to communicate with referring providers. Part of their practice is also in the ambulatory surgicenter, performing endoscopy and ambulatory operations.

To add an institution such as Three Rivers Community Hospital to a residency program, several requirements must be met. These requirements include (1) approval and appointment of all faculty, (2) assurance that policies were equivalent to those of the parent institution, (3) assurance that residents had access to our required educational conferences and that they have their own journal clubs and morbidity and mortality conferences, and (4) assurance of good supervision and evaluation of resident performance. The Accreditation Council for Graduate Medical Education (ACGME) work-hours regulations must be followed, and the ACGME competencies must be taught and evaluated. Residents must fulfill all medical staff obligations at the Three Rivers Community Hospital and must enter their cases in the surgical operative logs system. Having made sure that these requirements would be met, in May 2006, our program in Grants Pass was approved for a resident's experience to count as the fourth clinical year of training. After our first such resident completed the program and passed his American Board of Surgery certifying examination, we submitted our progress report to the Residency Review Committee in Surgery, and we were later approved for the second resident's experience to count as well.

Table 1
Specific learning objectives of the surgery residency program

Medical knowledge and patient care	The resident will demonstrate:
	1. Knowledge of the anatomy; pathophysiology; common modes of presentation; and appropriate treatment of common surgical emergencies and conditions in the fields of gynecology, orthopedic surgery, urology, otolaryngology, and genera and vascular surgery. They will demonstrate the ability to recognize these conditions on presentation and to describe and execute appropriate emergency treatment. These conditions specifically include the following:
	Gynecology: ectopic pregnancy; pelvic inflammatory disease; vaginal, uterine and cervical bleeding; acute pelvic pain; obstetric emergencies including indications for caesarean section; and management of adnexal masses and endometriosis when encountered at surgery.
	Orthopedic surgery: upper and lower extremity fractures and dislocations; spine fractures; evaluation of hand infections and injuries; and peripheral nerve compression.
	Urology: testicular torsion, priapism, testicular mass, renal mass, penile lesions, hematuria, and placement of the difficult Foley catheter and suprapubic catheter.
	Otolaryngology: facial and oral trauma; foreign body in airway, ear, and nose; epistaxis; dislocated jaw; peritonsillar abscess; and benign and malignant skin lesions.
	General and vascular surgery: the acute abdomen; acute cholecystitis and cholangitis; acute appendicitis; acute diverticulitis; upper and lower gastrointestinal hemorrhage; small and large intestinal obstruction; incarcerated hernias; ruptured abdominal aneurysm; application of Advanced Trauma Life Support principles of evaluation and management appropriate for a level III trauma center.
	2. The ability to access the appropriate medical literature relevant to the management of the conditions described earlier.
	3. Awareness of the indications for transfer of the patient to a tertiary center and the skill in communicating with the referral institution to accomplish safe patient care.

Practice-based learning and improvement	The resident will demonstrate: 1. The ability to analyze their own decisions and performance and describe areas of deficiency and strategies for improvement. 2. Use of the medical literature, both text and online, to select treatment strategies.
Interpersonal and communication skills	The resident will demonstrate: 1. The ability to effectively communicate care plans to patients, families, nurses, and other health care personnel. 2. Prompt and courteous response to the requests of staff. 3. The ability to work effectively with others as a member of the health care team.
Professionalism	The resident will demonstrate: 1. Responsiveness to the needs of patients and hospital staff. 2. Prompt and complete dictations and other medical documentation. 3. Respect, compassion, and integrity.
Systems-based practice	The resident will demonstrate: 1. Awareness of the limitations of their discipline and the appropriate interaction with other medical specialties to help in meeting the diverse needs of their patients. 2. Awareness of the need to transfer the patient to a tertiary institution for care when appropriate. 3. Attention to cost-effective care in ordering tests and planning interventions.

RESULTS

Ten residents have spent a year in Grants Pass to the present time. Six have completed their residency and have entered practice. Three entered and completed a fellowship after residency (1 in minimally invasive surgery, 1 in plastic surgery, and 1 in vascular surgery), and 3 entered practice directly after completing their residency. Two are practicing general surgery in a rural or international setting, whereas 3 more are in small but nonrural community practice in general surgery. Only 1 is practicing exclusively in a surgical specialty in an urban setting. These statistics compare favorably with those of the 55 other graduates from the same time period, none of whom is practicing general surgery in a rural setting and 39 (71%) of whom entered specialty fellowships.

LIMITATIONS

Because the residents who spend the year in Grants Pass are self-selected, we cannot suggest that our program has caused individuals to enter or consider rural surgical practice who were not already inclined to do so. However, that their experience reinforced their interest in rural practice is encouraging.

FUTURE DIRECTIONS

Although the total number of rural surgeons that the program has produced is modest as a result of few participants, the outcomes are promising and warrant continuation of the program. Other possibilities for the future involve adding other high-quality hospitals in small communities in our state that have expressed interest in partnering with our institution, to help expand the general surgical workforce for small and medium-sized communities. Because medical students at our institution already rotate to some of these settings for 5-week periods, the faculty may be receptive to having residents for shorter rotation lengths, thus providing more residents with some exposure to small community practice. Another option that we have considered but not yet implemented is a 1-year postresidency rural fellowship under mentorship of a surgeon or surgical group in a small community. The need for more general surgeons who are prepared and willing to serve rural communities is well recognized and growing. Based on our experience over the past 7 years, it remains our belief that residents will benefit from a training program that provides extensive exposure to procedures unique to a rural practice.

REFERENCES

1. Physician workforce in Oregon 2004: a snapshot. Oregon Health & Science University Center for Rural Health. Available at: http://www.ohsu.edu/oregonruralhealth. Accessed March 7, 2005.
2. Landercasper J, Bintz M, Cogbill TH, et al. Spectrum of general surgery in rural America. Arch Surg 1997;132:1239–40.
3. Heneghan SJ, Bordley J, Dietz PA, et al. Comparison of urban and rural general surgeons: motivations for practice location, practice patterns, and education requirements. J Am Coll Surg 2005;201:732–6.
4. Ritchie WP, Rhodes RS, Biester TW. Work loads and practice patterns of general surgeons in the United States, 1995–1997: a report from the American Board of Surgery. Ann Surg 1999;230:533–43.

Rural General Surgery Training: The Gundersen Lutheran Approach

Thomas H. Cogbill, MD, FACS[a,b,*], Benjamin T. Jarman, MD, FACS[a,b]

KEYWORDS

- Surgery residency • Rural surgery • Surgery training
- Practice management • Practice-based learning

The practice of general surgery in a rural location is alluring and challenging to interested individuals. The chance to perform a broad range of procedures, experience unparalleled independence, and immediately become a vital part of one's hospital and community are very attractive attributes. However, these joys are offset by professional isolation, inability to find call coverage, and difficulty keeping up with technological and intellectual advances in surgery. Clearly, training residents to adequately prepare for rural general surgery practice requires unique and innovative methods for promoting success in these settings, through development of the necessary skill sets, lifelong learning, and practice management knowledge. At Gundersen Lutheran, there has been a longstanding interest in training the rural general surgeon. The surgical residency program has been designed to address many of these issues in response to the institution's studies on the spectrum of procedures performed by rural surgeons,[1] the role of rural general surgeons functioning within trauma systems,[2,3] and the unique challenges of training rural surgeons.[4] This background, in conjunction with the geography and structure of Gundersen Lutheran, has made it an excellent place to prepare residents for rural general surgery.

GUNDERSEN LUTHERAN SETTING

Gundersen Lutheran is a multispecialty group practice established by Adolf Gundersen in 1891. In 2009, this fully integrated, physician-led health care system includes 453 physicians and 6159 employees working at the main campus in La Crosse, Wisconsin

[a] Surgery Residency, Gundersen Lutheran Medical Foundation, 1900 South Avenue, La Crosse, WI 54601, USA
[b] Surgery Residency, Gundersen Lutheran Health System, 1900 South Avenue, La Crosse, WI 54601, USA
* Corresponding author.
E-mail address: thcogbil@gundluth.org (T.H. Cogbill).

Surg Clin N Am 89 (2009) 1309–1312
doi:10.1016/j.suc.2009.07.006
0039-6109/09/$ – see front matter © 2009 Elsevier Inc. All rights reserved.

(population 50,266) and at 25 regional sites in 19 agricultural counties of Wisconsin, Iowa, and Minnesota. The Department of Surgery includes 14 full-time teaching faculty members in La Crosse and 9 rural general surgeons at 7 regional locations.

GUNDERSEN LUTHERAN SURGERY RESIDENCY

Gundersen Lutheran Medical Foundation has sponsored a 5-year surgical residency since 1974. At the most recent Accreditation Committee on Graduate Medical Education review by the Residency Review Committee for Surgery, a 5-year approval with commendation was received. The residency currently offers 2 categorical positions. Since the inception of the program, there have been 46 graduates, all of whom have achieved certification by the American Board of Surgery. On residency completion, 11 (24%) graduates have chosen postgraduate fellowships (2 additional graduates entered fellowships several years after having been in general surgery practice), whereas 35 (76%) have directly entered the practice of general surgery. Of those practicing general surgery, 23 (66%) have chosen to practice in towns with populations less than 10,000. Eight graduates currently practice in a teaching hospital.

STRONG CORE GENERAL SURGERY TRAINING

Our residents participate in a high-volume practice of general and minimally invasive surgery (MIS) during all 5 years of training. The average graduate completes more than 1200 major operations, including 200 basic and 110 advanced laparoscopic procedures. To assist with the acquisition of surgical technique, the Gundersen Lutheran Medical Foundation opened a dedicated surgical skills laboratory in 1995. Each month, the residents participate in a mandatory 3-hour technical skills session. All surgical residents complete 2 months on a high-volume endoscopy rotation, finishing with 150 colonoscopy and 50 upper gastrointestinal endoscopy procedures. Trauma and critical care education is emphasized throughout all 5 years of residency. Residents are primarily responsible for their own patients, admitted to intensive care units on every clinical rotation. Postgraduate year (PGY) 1 and PGY3 residents are exclusively assigned to the intensive care unit for 1 month to learn ventilator management, nutritional assessment, and invasive monitoring procedures. All PGY4 and PGY5 residents are trauma team leaders for resuscitations in the American College of Surgeons (ACS)-verified level II trauma center. All senior surgery residents are active Advanced Trauma Life Support (ATLS) instructors.

ADDITIONAL SKILL SETS

General surgery is the only surgical specialty that sponsors a residency, and a 1-year bariatric/MIS fellowship is the only postgraduate fellowship offered at Gundersen Lutheran. Therefore, surgical residents work one-on-one with attending staff from orthopedic surgery, neurosurgery, otolaryngology, plastic surgery, cardiothoracic surgery, and urology, when assigned to these services. As a result, resident graduates garner significant operative experience as surgeons in each of these specialty areas. In addition, the residency requires 2 months of obstetrics and gynecology during the third year of residency. Graduates complete more than 25 cesarean sections, 20 hysterectomies, and many gynecologic oncology cases. Residents interested in rural practice are encouraged to complete electives in plastic surgery and otolaryngology. Finally, comprehensive preoperative risk assessment and postoperative care of surgical patients are taught in an environment in which patient ownership and continuity of care are fostered in favor of immediate consultation for every medical condition encountered.

RURAL SURGERY ELECTIVES

Residents who demonstrate or develop an interest in rural general surgery are encouraged to select 1-month electives during PGY4 with busy Gundersen Lutheran regional surgeons who practice broad spectrum general surgery in Prairie du Chien, Wisconsin (population 6047), and Decorah, Iowa (population 7944). During these months the residents live in the community and are on call with their attending surgeons at the rural hospitals. They are responsible for all surgical patients, including their critical care and nutritional needs. They experience trauma care from a different perspective and are made aware of the rural surgeon's role in a small community hospital. Surgical volumes during these months include a large number of general surgery, obstetrics and gynecology, and endoscopic procedures. For residents who know in advance where they would like to practice rural surgery, electives have been arranged for several months at the rural hospital in which they intend to practice. This has allowed the resident to experience being fully immersed in rural surgery and to determine the additional skill sets that would be useful to acquire before joining that practice. Finally, an international elective rotation to a medically underserved nation has been established, in which residents perform a large number of common surgical procedures in an isolated setting.

PRACTICE-BASED LEARNING COMPONENTS

Academic excellence is paramount in the Gundersen Lutheran surgical residency. Attendance at weekly clinical conferences and basic science lectures and at monthly evidence-based journal clubs is mandatory. Before graduation, all residents are required to complete 2 publications in peer-reviewed journals and 2 presentations before learned societies. All these activities are focused on developing good habits for lifelong learning and professional poise for presentations. There is awareness that rural surgeons feel particularly vulnerable to "volume as a surrogate for quality" initiatives. The best defense for surgeons with low-to-moderate procedure volumes is ongoing knowledge of their own outcomes. All residents receive training in surgical case log analysis and are part of the institution's National Surgical Quality Improvement Program process. With a background in clinical research and quality initiatives, residency graduates are well prepared to support their practices with the prospective collection of outcomes data.

PRACTICE MANAGEMENT ELEMENTS

To better prepare graduates for the business side of surgical practice, Gundersen Lutheran has developed a curriculum of system-based practice topics. Lectures and practical exercises in coding and reimbursement, malpractice protection and defense preparation, contracts, and practice administration are interspersed throughout the year. For the past 20 years, clinical ethics conferences, under the direction of a doctoral-level medical ethicist, have been given every other month. Financial planning seminars are offered for residents and their spouses on an annual basis. Others have emphasized the importance of these activities during residency.[5]

RESPONSIBILITY TO GRADUATES

In an effort to mitigate the effects of professional isolation felt by rural general surgeons, the Gundersen Lutheran surgical residency engenders ongoing relationships with its graduates. Faculty members act as friendly resources with whom graduates can discuss difficult patient and administrative problems. The Gundersen

Lutheran Medical Foundation offers periodic continuing medical education programs to which the graduates are invited as speakers and participants. Several rural graduates return to La Crosse annually to teach a portion of an ATLS course or surgical skills laboratory. Some of the graduates have served as teaching faculty and mentors for a rural surgery elective. Having a large number of practicing rural surgery graduates has also provided a rich opportunity for research in surgical education.

SUMMARY

Many surgical residency programs define their success by the number of graduates who pursue competitive postgraduate fellowships or join university departments of surgery. The practice of general surgery in a rural hospital has its own unique set of formidable challenges and rich rewards. Gundersen Lutheran graduates who are willing to make this commitment are a source of equal pride.

REFERENCES

1. Landercasper J, Bintz M, Cogbill TH, et al. Spectrum of general surgery in rural America. Arch Surg 1997;132(5):494–6 [discussion: 496–8].
2. Ruby BJ, Cogbill TH, Gardner RS. Role of the rural general surgeon in a statewide trauma system: the Wyoming experience. Bull Am Coll Surg 2006;91(4):37–40.
3. Bintz M, Cogbill TH, Bacon J. Rural trauma care: role of the general surgeon. J Trauma 1996;41(3):462–4.
4. Cogbill TH. Training surgeons for rural America. Am Surg 2007;73(2):148–51.
5. Jones K, Lebron RA, Mangram A, et al. Practice management education during surgical residency. Am J Surg 2008;196(6):878–81 [discussion: 881–2].

Education of the Rural Surgeon: Experience from Tennessee

W. Heath Giles, MD[a], Joshua D. Arnold, MD[a], Thomas S. Layman, MD, FACS[b], Michael P. Sumida, MD, FACS[b], Preston W. Brown, MD, FACS[b], R. Phillip Burns, MD, FACS[a], Joseph B. Cofer, MD, FACS[a],*

KEYWORDS

• Rural surgery • Surgical endoscopy • General surgery training
• Surgical education • General surgeon role model

The department of surgery has seen a general trend toward specialization of faculty and also of resident rotations. In Chattanooga, our faculty of 32 attending surgeons includes only a small number of "traditional" general surgeons. In 1995, our surgical faculty was composed of 9 principal faculty surgeons, many of whom practiced "traditional" general surgery (including breast, vascular, gastrointestinal, and hernia surgeries) at Erlanger Medical Center, which is the main teaching hospital. By 2009, the faculty has grown to 32 surgeons, and most of them are specialized to some degree in any one area, for example, breast, vascular, or bariatric surgery. Our objective of resident training has always been to train competent general surgeons who are skilled, autonomous, and equipped to begin a full general surgery practice immediately out of residency. However, with the growing specialization and subspecialization in surgery, it is apparent that as present-day residents move from one specialty rotation to another, they get minimal exposure to role models who practice as our predecessors did or who practice as many surgeons do in nonacademic practice. Our rural surgery rotation fills this void with 3 additional faculty surgeons who practice in a rural setting.

In 2007, only 21% of graduating general surgeons nationally were planning to forgo fellowship training, a statistic that potentially worsens the existing shortage of general surgeons in the workforce.[1] This real and looming shortage of general surgeons threatens the existence of small rural hospitals, as these practitioners are relied on to provide surgical and endoscopic expertise that is critical to access for care for local

[a] Department of Surgery, University of Tennessee College of Medicine–Chattanooga, 979 East Third Street, Suite B401, Chattanooga, TN 37403, USA
[b] University of Tennessee College of Medicine–Chattanooga, McMinn Surgical Group, 719 Cook Drive, Suite 110, Athens, TN 37303, USA
* Corresponding author.
E-mail address: joe.cofer@erlanger.org (J.B. Cofer).

Surg Clin N Am 89 (2009) 1313–1319
doi:10.1016/j.suc.2009.07.005
surgical.theclinics.com
0039-6109/09/$ – see front matter © 2009 Elsevier Inc. All rights reserved.

patients and for economic viability of local hospitals. Rural communities often have a scarcity of specialists, and many of its citizens have neither the means nor the desire to travel to a surrounding larger city for such services. In addition, rural hospitals rely on surgical procedures for revenue, and reports suggest that each general surgeon is worth between 1 and 2.4 million dollars in annual revenue to the institution.[1]

Endoscopy has become a procedure dominated by gastroenterologists in most urban medical centers. Because most general surgery residency programs reside in urban locations, it is often difficult for surgical residents to meet the minimum case numbers required for endoscopy accreditation. More importantly, it is difficult to have the numbers and continuity of cases to feel adequately confident to incorporate this service into their practice. In a rural setting, the only endoscopist available is frequently the general surgeon, so the opportunity for endoscopic experience for the surgical resident in such a location is greater, assuming, that willing and competent faculty are available.

In an effort to define the scope of training in rural surgery, Burkholder and Cofer[2] surveyed program directors from 242 American surgery residency programs. Survey results indicated that although numerous articles have spoken for the development of a training track in rural surgery (either as a separate tract during residency or as a subspecialty), there is currently no consistent definition of what this curriculum should include. Only 36% of respondents reported having a rural surgery rotation, and programs were more likely to have such an experience as a fixed and prominent part of the curriculum if they believed training rural surgeons was a part of their mission. In Chattanooga, we feel this is a critical part of our mission.

Over a decade ago, we created a rotation that exposed residents to a thriving practice composed solely of traditional general surgeons in a rural location. Aside from the value of exposure to this career option, it was anticipated that resident participants would also be exposed to a rich experience in gastrointestinal endoscopy. The rural surgery rotation has become our predominant endoscopy rotation.

The purpose of this article is to document the experience of the rural surgery rotation provided by the Department of Surgery of the University of Tennessee College of Medicine–Chattanooga (UTCOMC). Athens, Tennessee is located 50 miles northeast of the primary teaching hospital for our training program and boasts 2 hospitals— Athens Regional Medical Center and Woods Memorial Hospital. There are 5 practicing general surgeons in Athens. Three of these board-certified surgeons practice together; they are all graduates of the UTCOMC surgical program (1995, 2000, and 2002) and serve as adjunct clinical professors with UTCOMC. The resident rotation is scheduled during the third year of training and is 3 months in length, and during this time, the resident has no other responsibilities in the program. The resident has the option to commute or dwell in Athens at no charge.

METHODS

An anonymous survey was administered to all current residents in our program who completed the rural surgery rotation between July 2006 and December 2008 (N = 12) (**Table 1**). The survey consisted of 13 questions about the rotation in standard 5-item Likert format. The 5 possible responses ranged from "strongly disagree," which was assigned a value of 1, to "strongly agree," which was assigned a value of 5. All responses for each question were averaged to yield a mean score. In addition, the 3-month case logs of authors H.G. and J.A. were compiled to illustrate the quantity and variety of cases performed during the rotation (**Table 2**).

Table 1
Resident experience survey

Athens Experience	Strongly Agree	Agree	Neutral	Disagree	Strongly Disagree	Scale
The Athens experience was valuable for my surgical education	11	1	0	0	0	4.9
The rotation was fun and educational	9	3	0	0	0	4.8
The endoscopy experience of Athens was beneficial	12	0	0	0	0	5.0
I feel prepared to incorporate endoscopy into my practice	12	0	0	0	0	5.0
The general surgery experience was beneficial	10	2	0	0	0	4.8
Attendings in Athens took an interest in my education	9	3	0	0	0	4.8
I left the rotation with a positive opinion of rural general surgery	7	4	1	0	0	4.5
I was considering rural surgery as a career option before my rotation	4	0	3	3	2	3.1
My experience caused me to consider rural general surgery as a career	6	0	2	2	2	3.5
Work hours were reasonable and work-hour restrictions were followed	9	3	0	0	0	4.8
I wish I had more time to spend on the Athens rotation	8	0	2	2	0	4.2
Residents are given ample autonomy on the Athens rotation	7	5	0	0	0	4.6
Resident housing accommodations were adequate	7	5	0	0	0	4.6

Table 2
Average case numbers for authors H.G. and J.A.

Endoscopy	Case Numbers
EGD	40
Colonoscopy	81
General surgery	
Laparoscopic cholecystectomy	44
Colectomy	10
Ventral hernia repair	9
Inguinal hernia repair	8
Appendectomy	7
Thyroidectomy	5
Hemorrhoidectomy	3
Tonsillectomy	3
Laparoscopic Nissen	2
Circumcision	2
Partial mastectomy	2
Nephrectomy	2
Tunneled central venous catheter insertion	2
Miscellaneous	
Stereotactic breast biopsy	
Parathyroidectomy	
Muscle biopsy	
Port (Port-A-Cath) removal	
Skin graft	
Lung lobectomy	
Removal of skin lesion	
Enterolysis	
Incision and drainage of abscess	
Oophorectomy	
Modified radical mastectomy	
Central venous line	
Small bowel resection	
Toe amputation	
Vasectomy	
Paracentesis	
Tube thoracostomy	

Actual numbers were assigned to the most commonly performed procedures. Miscellaneous cases were included to illustrate the variety of cases performed.

RESULTS

Residents reported the rural surgery rotation to be a highly valuable experience, with a mean score of 4.9. They felt that the rotation was fun and educational, with a mean score of 4.8. Work-hour restrictions were followed, and housing accommodations were adequate, with mean scores of 4.8 and 4.6, respectively. Residents felt that faculty attendings took an interest in their education and that they were given ample autonomy, with mean scores of 4.8 and 4.6, respectively. A positive response was elicited with regards to wishing that more time was allocated to this experience, with a mean score of 4.2.

The strongest positive response (mean score of 5.0) was found in the endoscopy experience evaluation, in which residents found the endoscopy experience to be beneficial and felt prepared to incorporate endoscopy into their practice. The general surgery experience exclusive of endoscopy was also felt to be strongly beneficial, with a mean score of 4.8.

The largest deviation in responses concerned items pertaining to rural surgery as a career. Residents reported considering rural surgery as a career before the rotation, with a mean score of 3.1. Four residents agreed or strongly agreed with the response "considering rural surgery as a career" (item 8, **Table 1**), 5 disagreed or strongly disagreed, and 3 were neutral. Residents finished the rotation with a positive opinion of rural surgery, with a mean score of 4.5. This positive opinion led to an increase in the mean score of residents now considering rural surgery as a career (item 9, **Table 1**) to 3.5. Six residents agreed or strongly agreed, 4 disagreed or strongly disagreed, and 2 were neutral.

On average, residents will perform 238 cases during their 3-month rural surgery rotation. Of these cases, 51% (121/238) are endoscopic procedures and 49% (117/238) are operative general surgery cases.

DISCUSSION
Endoscopy

In many rural general surgery practices, endoscopy is an integral part of daily practice. One report demonstrated that rural surgeons perform flexible endoscopy at a much higher rate than their nonrural counterparts.[3] An endoscopic skill set is essential to step into such a practice where the diagnosis and treatment of common gastrointestinal complaints is a mainstay of general surgery experience. The Residency Review Committee (RRC) requires a minimum of 50 colonoscopy procedures for graduating chiefs. We have found that endoscopy experience at the main teaching hospital in Chattanooga is more difficult to obtain, is at times sporadic, and could leave the resident lacking in sufficient repetition necessary to confidently acquire these skills.

During the Athens rotation, endoscopy procedures are typically performed at an outpatient surgery center. A generous schedule and a rapid turnover of endoscopic cases provide the resident an opportunity to master the skills through repetition. Residents perform an average of 81 colonoscopies and 40 esophagogastroduodenoscopies (EGDs) during this 3-month rotation, which more than meets the RRC minimum requirements. This rotation also allows for practice with therapeutic endoscopy, including thermal coagulation and injection of upper gastrointestinal bleeding, and balloon dilatation of esophageal and pyloric strictures. These latter cases are usually performed at 1 of the 2 local hospitals where the surgical faculty practices.

Aside from procedure-related experience, office time is dedicated to the evaluation and treatment of common gastroenterologic pathologies, such as peptic ulcer disease, gastric polyps, helicobacter pylori, diverticulosis, constipation, chronic diarrhea, colon polyps, and general colon cancer screening and treatment.

General Surgery

The practice of a surgeon in a major metropolitan medical center often differs greatly from that of one in a rural setting. Surgeons in more urban centers tend to focus their practice on specific diseases or areas of subspecialized expertise and therefore can refer problems and cases to associates or other colleagues with more specialized training. In a rural setting, the general surgeon remains the surgical provider for a vast array of disease processes because the specialist is no longer just down the hall. This dichotomy frequently gives surgical residents without a rural experience a skewed perspective of what a general surgeon is, and can be, and underestimates the importance and pleasure of diversity of practice and educational opportunity available.

During a typical Athens rotation, it is common for our residents to get experience not only with typical gastrointestinal surgery but also with "specialty" procedures. On average, they perform 117 general surgery cases during the 3-month rotation. Our rural surgeon faculty often perform cases in otolaryngology (tonsillectomy), endocrine surgery (thyroidectomy, parathyroidectomy), gynecology (oophorectomy, hysterectomy), urology (nephrectomy, vasectomy, circumcision), colorectal surgery (colectomy, APR, hemorrhoidectomy) and breast surgery (mastectomy, stereotactic biopsy). The variety experienced is illustrated in **Table 2**. Although endoscopy is the major procedural focus of this rotation, almost half (49%) of the 238 cases are operative. It is important to realize that this diversity of practice can still be seen in many rural practices, and this type of career can be very exciting and rewarding.

Duty Hours/Office Experience

In compliance with the RRC regulations regarding work-hour restrictions, residents on the rural rotation typically work Monday to Friday, from 7 AM to 5 PM. Call is taken from home and is 1 day per week and 2 weekends per month. The general experience with call in this setting is much different from typical call at our major center. Surgical emergencies tend to be less common in a rural community because of a smaller population size. Major medical centers, such as ours in Chattanooga, are tertiary referral centers and therefore serve a much larger area. Call in Athens is home call and rarely ends as a totally sleepless night, whereas Chattanooga call is in-house and often a full second work shift, where the resident is busy the entire night. In making career choices, it is valuable to understand that all call nights are not created equal and that, on average, call in a rural setting tends to be less intense.

The 3 rural faculty surgeons hold office hours in the afternoon from Monday to Thursday. Residents are expected to participate with each attending's office at least once per week. Although the overall sentiment is a preference for being in the operating room, the office experience is an opportunity to follow an individual through the initial office visit, the operating room, and postoperative care, whereas there is less opportunity for door-to-door exposure at the tertiary center institution.

Housing and Funding

Housing is provided for residents who choose to stay in Athens for the duration of the rotation. The faculty group in Athens purchased a house for the resident's use. This home is provided free of charge and is large enough to accommodate the resident's spouse and children if they desire. Athens is also close enough to Chattanooga to allow for daily commutes. No extra malpractice coverage is necessary because the rotation is in the state of Tennessee, and residents are under the supervision of University of Tennessee, Department of Surgery faculty and subsequently have the same coverage as residents on the main campus. Residents receive their scheduled monthly salary from UTCOMC, as the local dean allows this loss of 1 full-time equivalent Graduate Medical Education (FTE GME)medical funding because of the immense educational value of the rotation.

Resident Experience

The rural surgery rotation is well received, and residents perceive it to be a valuable addition to their general surgery and endoscopy training. The rotation prepares our residents to perform basic endoscopic procedures, and all surveyed residents have reported that now they feel prepared to incorporate endoscopy into their practice. This is important not only because there is a shortage of rural surgeons but also because a large percentage of surgeons in current rural surgical practice believe that their endoscopy training experience in residency was inadequate.[3] We agree with previous publications that programs dedicated to training rural surgeons should provide more experience in endoscopy, and this rotation is our primary modality for achieving that goal.[4,5]

In the opinion of the Chattanooga faculty, the residents return from Athens more "seasoned." This rotation gives the residents a great deal of autonomy and allows them to act as an individual while having appropriate supervision.

Most residents leave Athens with a positive opinion of rural surgery. The survey shows a modest increase from 3.1 to 3.5 in pre- and postrotation plans to pursue a career in rural surgery. Also, the number of neutral responders decreased from 3 to 2. Although this survey contains small numbers, it supports previous studies, which indicate that exposure to the rural environment can help residents decide whether to enter rural practice or not.[6,7]

SUMMARY

Our rural surgery rotation is considered to be of high educational value by our residents, and it has become the backbone of our surgical endoscopy training. In addition, residents on this rotation have enhanced autonomy in other areas of surgical care, and they return to the main campus more accomplished and confident.

Most importantly, residents are heavily and intimately exposed over a 3-month rotation to true rural general surgeons who serve as role models. They gain additional information about this practice type, which allows them to compare the inner city, academic teaching hospital physician's practice with the rural surgeon's practice. A more informed decision can then be made about their future career paths.

REFERENCES

1. Cofer JB, Burns RP. The developing crisis in the national general surgery workforce. J Am Coll Surg 2008;206:790–7.
2. Burkholder HC, Cofer JB. Rural surgery training: a survey of program directors. J Am Coll Surg 2007;204:416–21.
3. Zuckerman R, Doty B, Bark K, et al. Rural versus non-rural differences in surgeon performed endoscopy: results of a national survey. Am Surg 2007;73:903–5.
4. Hunter JG, Deveney KE. Training the rural surgeon: a proposal. Bull Am Coll Surg 2003;88:13–7.
5. Reynolds FD, Goudas L, Zuckerman RS, et al. A rural, community-based program can train surgical residents in advanced laparoscopy. J Am Coll Surg 2003;197:620–3.
6. Asher EF, Martin LF, Richardson JD, et al. Rural rotations for senior surgical residents. Arch Surg 1984;119:1120–4.
7. Doty B, Heneghan S, Gold M, et al. Is a broadly based surgical residency program more likely to place graduates in rural practice? World J Surg 2006;30:2089–93.

Bassett Healthcare Rural Surgery Experience

David C. Borgstrom, MD, FACS*, Steven J. Heneghan, MD, FACS

KEYWORDS

- Surgical education • Subspecialty training • Rural surgery
- General surgery training • Mithoefer fellowship

The Mary Imogene Bassett Hospital in Cooperstown, New York was named in honor of a physician who devoted herself generously to the sick and unfortunate of Cooperstown and the surrounding countryside. Dr Bassett died in 1922, but her passion for the health care of her rural neighbors led to the establishment of a hospital in her name by a group of physicians from New York City. Local philanthropy and a commitment from Columbia University established a rural academic teaching hospital with dual missions of patient care and education.

The training of surgical residents has been part of the Bassett education mission for more than 50 years. The surgical training at Bassett is naturally broader than in many university settings. A recent survey showed that nearly 70% of its graduates who practice general surgery remain in a rurally designated area. Factors that lead to this include the rural location and the broad experience of the training program due to the lack of competing surgical subspecialty training programs. Today, as training paradigms evolve and work hour limitations affect flexibility and opportunities in many general surgery programs, there is a greater need and focus on broad-based general surgery training. Bassett has historically emphasized education, with the health care needs of rural America and the rural health care workforce in mind.

The Mithoefer Center for Rural Surgery was developed out of a recognized need for ongoing evaluation, investigation, and educational support for surgical care in rural America. It is named for Dr James Mithoefer, a surgeon on staff at Bassett in the 1950s and 1960s. In addition to his general surgery training, he received additional training in orthopedics and plastic surgery. He was a dedicated teacher. He established the first tumor registry in the upstate New York area. In 1963, he died tragically from complications due to multiple yellow jacket stings. His family has memorialized him through the Robert Keeler Foundation, by providing the funding needed to launch the Center for Rural Surgery named in his honor.

Mithoefer Center for Rural Surgery, Department of Surgery, Bassett Healthcare, 1 Atwell Road, Cooperstown, NY 13326, USA
* Corresponding author.
E-mail address: david.borgstrom@bassett.org (D.C. Borgstrom).

Surg Clin N Am 89 (2009) 1321–1323
doi:10.1016/j.suc.2009.07.011
0039-6109/09/$ – see front matter © 2009 Elsevier Inc. All rights reserved.

surgical.theclinics.com

Although 25% of Americans live in rural areas, only about 12% of physicians practice in those rural settings. This is especially true of surgeons; it is estimated that only 10% of general surgeons currently practice in rural environments, although some forecast the number needed to adequately care for rural America to be close to 19%. Along with primary care physicians, general surgeons are a crucial component of rural health care teams. The rural general surgeon provides necessary surgical services, trauma care, and critical care in small hospitals and various other surgical subspecialty areas, including endoscopy. The surgeon is at the core of financial stability in small rural hospitals. The Mithoefer Center for Rural Surgery was established in 2004 to confront these problems. It is committed to developing comprehensive solutions that benefit rural citizens, rural surgeons, and rural hospitals alike.

Rural surgery experience falls into 3 categories: undergraduate, graduate, and postgraduate. The educational setting is a rural small town with a population of approximately 2200 people. It is a tertiary care referral center with broad-based surgical experience. However, it provides this opportunity in a small rural community, which is ideal for those interested in rural health care to understand and appreciate small-town life.

In an attempt to expose younger students to the nature of rural health care careers, the "Shadow a Surgeon Program" has been developed. High school and undergraduate college students may spend from 2 days to 2 weeks with one of our surgeons or another health care provider to explore their interest in a health care career. To date, 30 students have participated in the program. For medical students, there is a specific fourth-year rural surgery elective, with students spending time on the main campus in Cooperstown and in the smaller, more remote settings where surgical care is provided and surgical patients are initially seen. The developing clinical campus in partnership with Columbia University will open in 2011, providing a comprehensive exposure to broad-based medical and surgical experiences in a rural setting. Students begin their medical career at Columbia University in New York City for 18 months, then complete their medical school education in Cooperstown.

The general surgery training program currently finishes 2 categorical chief residents, with a recently approved increase in complement of 3. There are no competing fellowships or subspecialty residencies; therefore, the residents get significant exposure to the broad-based categories of general surgery, including a significant experience with endoscopy; ear, nose, and throat (ENT); plastic and hand surgery; and obstetrics and gynecology (OB/GYN). There are dedicated rural surgery electives for junior residents, and our senior residents have an opportunity to spend 6 weeks in Saranac Lake, New York, in a broad-based surgical practice in the Adirondack Mountains, away from the main Cooperstown campus. Our intent is to show not only the broad scope of rural practice but also the appeal of a truly rural lifestyle.

Through the Center for Rural Surgery, the Mithoefer Fellowship in Rural Surgery was established. The intent is to provide an opportunity for board-certified or board-eligible surgeons who feel a personal need for more experience and exposure to the surgical subspecialties that would better enable them to provide care for their local communities. The general surgery training program at Bassett in Cooperstown has no competing subspecialty residents, allowing opportunities for fellows to gain exposure without being in direct competition or conflict with the resident experience.

Fellows have the opportunity to spend dedicated time in various surgical subspecialty areas and in the endoscopy suite, to enhance their personal skills in a needs-based program specifically designed for the practice setting they have in mind. It has evolved into more of a continuing professional development experience. To date, 7 fellows have completed Mithoefer Fellowships. They spent an average of 7 weeks in training. Three had plans to go on to international or missionary work, with 4 planning to go into practice in a rural setting. Four came specifically for more endoscopy experience, with the fellows performing approximately 50 endoscopy cases, both upper and lower. Three had broad-based subspecialty surgical interests, including ENT, plastic surgery, hand surgery, and OB/GYN, and 1 focused his time directly on urology. Flexibility allows the tailoring of experience directly to the needs of the fellow.

This is only one of many models intended to address the issues of surgical care for rural America. There are many opportunities to obtain additional training and expertise in endoscopy and subspecialty areas needed to be a well-prepared, broad-based rural surgeon. The experience of living and working in a small community is critical. It allows a real-life experience for those seemingly interested in surgery in small-town America. The rural setting lifestyle is valued by the students, residents, and fellows alike. It provides an ideal setting to recognize the specific nuances of small-town American life, with a high-quality education and surgical experience.

FURTHER READINGS

Heneghan SJ, Bordley J, Dietz PA, et al. Comparison of urban and rural general surgeons: motivations for practice location, practice patterns, and education requirements. J Am Coll Surg 2005;201(5):732–6.

Zuckerman R, Doty B, Bark K, et al. Rural versus non-rural differences in surgeon performed endoscopy: results of a national survey. Am Surg 2007;73(9):903–5.

Zuckerman R, Doty B, Gold M, et al. General surgery programs in small rural New York State hospitals: a pilot survey of hospital administrators. J Rural Health 2006;22(4):339–42.

Chappel A, Zuckerman RS, Finlayson SRG. Small rural hospitals and high risk surgery: how would regionalization affect surgical volume and hospital revenue? J Am Coll Surg 2006;203(5):599–604.

Doty B, Heneghan S, Gold M, et al. Is a broadly based surgical residency program more likely to place graduates in rural practice? World J Surg 2006;30(12): 2089–93.

Reynolds F, Goudas L, Zuckerman RS, et al. A rural, community-based program can train surgical residents in advanced laparoscopy. J Am Coll Surg 2003;197(4): 620–3.

Rural Surgery: The Australian Experience

Martin H. Bruening, BMBS, MS[a,b],*, Guy J. Maddern, MB, BS, PhD, MS[a]

KEYWORDS

- Australia • Rural surgical workforce
- Undergraduate education • Provincial hospitals
- General surgery

Australia, by virtue of its demographic and geographic characteristics, has a long history of rural surgery (**Fig. 1**). The majority of the Australian population resides in the major state capital cities, but a significant proportion live in nonmetropolitan regions. In Queensland, New South Wales, and Victoria, large provincial towns have allowed group general surgical practices to evolve and provide a wide range of surgical services to the community. The remaining states have regional centers, but do not have the same population base as their eastern states counterparts. For the majority of these smaller regional centers, the surgical service delivery is provided by either solo or two-person surgical practices. The smaller towns have traditionally been the domain of the general practitioner, many of whom provided excellent surgical service, both in emergency and elective procedures. Visiting surgeons would often supplement the surgical services in the smaller towns. In Western Australia, the University Department of Surgery at Queen Elizabeth II Medical Center in Perth has provided a visiting surgical service to the smaller rural communities, undertaking regular visits and operating sessions.[1] A specialist surgical outreach service has also been specifically designed for improving access to specialist care for remote Aboriginal communities in the Northern Territory.[2] In terms of the subspecialties, few provincial centers have been large enough to allow for resident urologists; ophthalmologists; and ears, nose, and throat or plastic surgeons. Traditionally, these services have been provided on a regular visiting basis.

Given the relative lack of access to the various subspecialties, many general surgeons of the past developed a wide range of skills encompassing procedures normally the domain of their subspecialty colleagues. For example, Australia has a high rate of skin cancer in the population and most rural general surgeons, by necessity, became adept at complex plastic surgery to serve their respective communities.

[a] Department of Surgery, University of Adelaide, The Queen Elizabeth Hospital, Adelaide, Woodville Road, Woodville 5011, South Australia, Australia
[b] University of South Australia/University of Adelaide Spencer Gulf Rural Health School, Whyalla Campus, Nicholson Avenue, Whyalla Norrie, South Australia 5608, Australia
* Corresponding author. Department of Surgery, University of Adelaide, The Queen Elizabeth Hospital, Adelaide, Woodville Road, Woodville 5011, South Australia, Australia.
E-mail address: martin.bruening@adelaide.edu.au (M.H. Bruening).

Surg Clin N Am 89 (2009) 1325–1333
doi:10.1016/j.suc.2009.07.004
0039-6109/09/$ – see front matter Crown Copyright © 2009 Elsevier Inc. All rights reserved.
surgical.theclinics.com

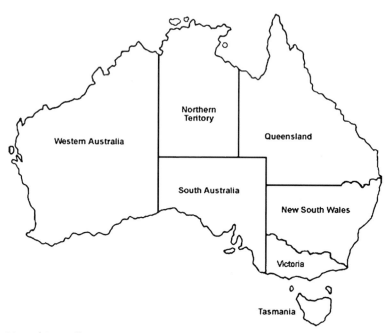

Fig. 1. Map of Australia.

One of the draw cards for surgeons to venture to the country has been the diversity of the surgery that can be performed, both on an elective and emergency basis.[3,4] Road trauma and farming accidents have been a leading source of emergency theater cases for rural general surgeons.[5] Whereas the Royal Flying Doctor Service (RFDS) and other aeromedical retrieval services have provided a safety net to the rural communities, situations continually arise where the local surgeon is called upon to stabilize the patient before transfer to a tertiary center.

Over the past 30 years, many factors have lead to an increased examination of rural health care delivery. A significant drift of population away from the smaller towns has resulted in many local hospitals closing the operating theater suite. With the passage of time, the skills of the general practitioner and nursing staff have also been lost and, currently, a major issue is the growing problem of a declining rural medical workforce. Community expectations have also increased, placing pressure on the general practitioner who may not feel comfortable performing certain (or any) surgical procedures. Opportunities do exist for general practitioners to undertake surgical terms in tertiary institutions, but these are limited in number and more importantly may not provide the practitioner with the particular skill set they are seeking.[6]

The Royal Australasian College of Surgeons (RACS) has formally recognized the need to assist individuals with an interest in rural surgery and subsequently established the rural surgical training program.[7] While the program essentially represents the general surgical program, flexibility exists for trainees to pursue a particular subspecialty interest that may be of benefit to community where they intend to establish their practice. The scheme has been in place for over 10 years and resulted in trainees becoming rural surgeons.

The medical workforce issues have also influenced surgical services, especially in the regional centers where one or two surgeons have worked. Recent reports have illustrated that a significant proportion of Australia's surgical workforce is aging and this is nowhere more acute than in the rural regions.[8,9] As with the general practitioner, there is a seeming lack of interest in young surgeons venturing to the country and, despite the efforts of the RACS and the rural surgical training program, a distinct shortage remains. The reasons for not leaving the metropolitan area are many and varied, but several factors are constant. Professional isolation, the amount of on-call, spousal employment opportunities, and schooling for children are the issues most often listed.[3,10] The difficulty encountered in procuring a locum surgeon to provide relief for resident surgeons has been eased by the establishment of a locum specialist service (RACS), but the number of city-based surgeons willing to provide cover for their country colleagues remains limited.

As the next generation of medical graduates continues to address the work–life balance, the chances of an upsurge in graduates, both general practice and specialist, venturing to the rural areas appear minimal. The increasing feminization of the work-force may also have an effect on workforce delivery. One suggested model of surgical service delivery is to link a regional hospital post with a tertiary hospital such that if a newly qualified specialist went to a rural post for a 2-year tenure, guarantees of a position at the principle teaching hospital upon their return to the city would be given.[11]

The ability of a rural surgeon to deliver effective service is also dependent on the infrastructure of the relevant hospital. It has only been in the last decade that all of the major regional centers in the Spencer Gulf region of South Australia have acquired CT scanners, a radiological service considered essential by surgeons. An anesthetic service is also essential and, in many rural locations, this has been provided with great skill by general practitioners. Intensive care facilities are readily available only in the larger eastern state population centers, and this may be a limiting factor in a local general surgeon's willingness to perform complex cases in the smaller centers existing elsewhere in Australia.

The issue of on-call arrangements for emergency cover is also difficult to resolve. A major report on Australia's surgical workforce, done 10 years ago, suggested that for a regional center to have a resident surgical service, a population base large enough to sustain two general surgeons was required.[9] This would still translate to an on call rotation of 1:2, not allowing for time taken for leave or professional development. It is difficult to believe that the current generation of graduates, raised on a roster where time off is guaranteed, would embrace a busy 1:2 roster on becoming a consultant. This is not to say that work–life balance is unimportant, but rather to highlight the fact that for surgical services to continue in some rural locations, two replacements may be required for every single retirement. A more recent report into specialist rural services has recommended that on-call is performed on a 1 in 4 rota.[12] Implementa-tion into the rural hospitals of the safe working hour policies currently enforced for junior medical staff in the metropolitan setting would have major ramifications in terms of constructing emergency call rosters with the current workforce shortages.[13] For example, if a surgeon operated on a patient at 2 AM as a matter of emergency, indus-trial law may prevent them from consulting or operating that morning. If the surgeon chooses to ignore this ruling, any possible adverse events that occur subsequently may have serious legal ramifications.

Mention has already been made of one significant effort, that of the RACS, to address surgical shortages in the rural regions. In recent years, the Australian government has established several rural medical schools with the intention of producing, not only competent and well-trained graduates, but also looking toward the future by encouraging medical undergraduates to consider rural careers by exposing them to positive rural experiences. It has long been recognized that the two factors which influence an individual to consider a rural practice are a rural upbringing and an early exposure to rural medicine as an undergraduate.[14,15]

South Australia is a predominantly urban-centered state with approximately 75% of the population residing within a 100 km radius of the capital, Adelaide (**Fig. 2**). In terms of size, the area involved is approximately the size of Texas (**Fig. 3**). A significant number of people live in the rural sector, mostly clustered in several regional centers. Given the distances involved in travel to Adelaide, surgical services have developed within the regional centers that use the traditional model of a resident surgeon or surgeons providing 24-hour coverage, 365 days per year. This model has largely remained unchallenged as the accepted mode of surgical service delivery and, whereas it has merit in the eastern states of Australia where larger regional centers are able to attract a number of surgeons, the smaller centers in South Australia have traditionally functioned on a solo or, at best, two-person practice. The rural surgeons in South Australia have managed to provide an excellent standard of surgical service for many years. Inevitably, however, retirements and reluctance by younger surgeons to venture outside of the metropolitan area has demanded a rethink concerning service delivery.

Over the past decade, the University of Adelaide has developed new models of surgical provision in several of the regional centers. These models take on the responsibility for providing the surgeons to the town to either support existing resident surgeons or provide 365 days per year coverage for the town.[16]

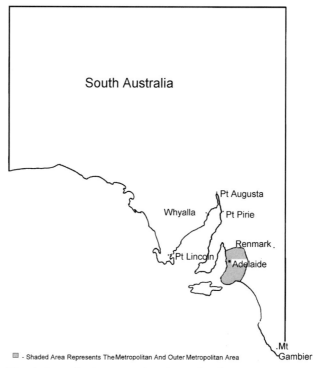

☐ - Shaded Area Represents The Metropolitan And Outer Metropolitan Area

Fig. 2. Map of South Australia demonstrating the regional centers.

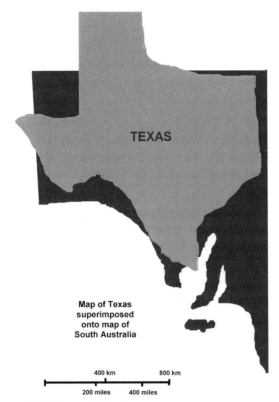

**Map of Texas
superimposed
onto map of
South Australia**

```
400 km          800 km
├────────┼────────┤
   200 miles   400 miles
```

Fig. 3. Comparison of South Australia to Texas.

MODEL 1: PORT AUGUSTA

Port Augusta is a major regional center at the top of the Spencer Gulf, some 300 km from Adelaide by road. There is a resident population of 15,000 with an additional outreach population of 13,000 covering an area the size of France. This area of the state is currently experiencing a mining resources boom and conservative estimates are that the population will increase significantly over the next decade. The RFDS has a base at Port Augusta and services the far north of the state. Given the population numbers, the RFDS base, and the fact that Port Augusta is located at the junction of several major highways, a 24-hour surgical service is required.

Visiting surgeons from the Department of Surgery at the University of Adelaide provide a 7 days per week roster covering the town for consultations, surgical procedures, and emergency coverage. Complex cases are referred to Adelaide to a teaching hospital served by the surgeon who is in town at the time. In this way, continuity of care is ensured for the complex and difficult cases, but the more straightforward and routine work is performed on a rotational basis. This program has been in place for over 14 years and provides a consistent and sustained service to the town without any interruptions of care. Even when situations of sudden illness for the surgeon in the town occur, a replacement surgeon is provided within 12 hours. In this way, there is no risk to surgical cover for the community.

The program is well embraced and has expanded to provide weekend coverage for Whyalla and Port Pirie, two communities approximately 1 hour away from Port

Augusta. This has enabled the resident surgeon in Port Pirie to have weekend relief and to maintain an on-call roster that is more acceptable, rather than perpetuating an unreasonable 1:1 roster with the consequent burn-out factor. In essence, the resource that is being placed in Port Augusta is gaining maximal use across the weekend coverage period where, although the number of emergency cases is relatively low, the need for a fresh surgeon is essential. It is for this reason that the beginning of the roster commences on the weekend so that the surgeon is not already reaching the end of a busy week, but rather is at the commencement of their rotation.

In addition to these initiatives, this placement of the surgical workforce allows the positioning of a surgical trainee in Port Augusta, which greatly enhances the teaching opportunities and almost certainly influences the quality of surgical care. In addition, medical students' opportunities to undertake a rural surgical term are expanded with this model. The Port Augusta term remains extremely popular and is widely sought after. This is undoubtedly because the students are exposed to a number of surgeons who are eager to teach for their week in Port Augusta. From the surgeon's perspective, the fatigue associated with the teaching of medical students on a regular basis is avoided because of the short-term nature of the rotation. The rural surgical undergraduate terms have been shown to be as effective as the tertiary hospital terms in providing a sound surgical education, with rural students consistently excelling in final examinations.[17] The overall experience of the rural terms have been subjectively rated by the students as being of great value, with access to a broad range of surgical cases and conditions not seen within specialized tertiary hospital units.[18,19]

MODEL 2: MOUNT GAMBIER

Mount Gambier is South Australia's largest regional center with a population of 25,000 and an outeach area of 80,000 people. The town is 600 km by road from Adelaide. Several years ago, three general surgeons were recruited to the town and supported with close links to the University of Adelaide—in particular, The Queen Elizabeth Hospital. Locum cover and weekend support is provided by the metropolitan surgeons and a weekly ward round is conducted by video link between the two hospitals. During the ward round, difficult cases are presented and discussed. In addition to these support mechanisms, complex cases requiring extensive tertiary hospital infrastructure, such as major esophageal and pancreatic resections are performed in Adelaide, with the Mount Gambier surgeon offered the option of participating in the procedure. The general surgeons work under the direct supervision and management of the Director of Surgery at The Queen Elizabeth Hospital, who manages the political and professional issues that arise in their practice on their behalf. Discussions between the Mount Gambier hospital management and the Director of Surgery at The Queen Elizabeth Hospital occur to ensure that the appropriate work environment is maintained and enhanced for surgeons.

As a result of the well-supported surgical service delivery in Mount Gambier, outreach programs to other hospitals within the region are being developed with the resident surgeons providing surgical care.

Owing to the commitment of the surgeons, a surgical trainee has been placed in Mount Gambier for the first time and it is anticipated that further training opportunities will arise over the ensuing years, given the abundance of surgical cases and exposure to a broad range of general surgery.[20] As is the case with Port Augusta, medical students have eagerly sought the chance to undertake their surgical terms in Mount Gambier and this is a testament to the surgeons involved in all levels in the town.

MODEL 3: PORT LINCOLN

Port Lincoln is designated as a remote town, being almost 800 km by road from Adelaide. The town is the center for the Eyre Peninsula and has an immediate population of 15,000 with an outreach population of 15,000. For many years, this entire area has been serviced by a solo surgeon, providing an outstanding contribution to the community. However, obtaining leave for recreation and professional development has been difficult. The University of Adelaide has developed a program whereby a metropolitan surgeon travels to Port Lincoln on a monthly basis for a week at a time. On one of the rotations, the visiting surgeon will provide peer support with assistance at operations and second opinions in addition to their own independent operating. The following monthly rotation will involve taking over complete responsibility for the surgical practice. Using this model allows the resident surgeon to have a guaranteed week off in every seven and remove the emergency cover load, one week in four. The program commenced in May 2008 and, as it develops, it is envisaged that a trainee will be placed in Port Lincoln to provide additional support to the resident surgeon and, at the same time, gain invaluable surgical training and experience.

SUMMARY

The model of care described for Port Augusta has been in existence for 14 years and been expanded to encompass Whyalla and Port Pirie over the past 6 years. Mount Gambier has been successful for the last 3 years and it is anticipated that the initiative proposed for Port Lincoln will provide a sustainable and robust method of surgical support.

These models of care can be applied to similar rural settings within Australia if there is a commitment from the larger institutions, often with academic links, to organize and provide the opportunities. There is no doubt that the surgeons who become involved in these programs develop a much greater appreciation of the challenges of rural surgery and enjoy the clinical opportunity. On the whole, it has been possible, once they have been introduced to the concept, to have a steady stream of recruits to continue to staff the positions. It has been noted that a number of the surgeons providing this service are of the recent generation of graduating Fellows from the College. Another interesting variable is that a number of more mature surgeons, as they wish to pull back from their private practice in the cities, have taken up the opportunity to practice in the country under these arrangements. It provides them with the ability to provide a service without having to uproot their family and alter their domestic situation.

The impact these models have on providing surgical training at both under- and postgraduate levels cannot be underestimated. For many years, local medical schools did not send students outside of the metropolitan region to undertake surgical rotations. By providing a consistent surgical service in Port Augusta and supporting the resident surgeons in other centers, the true value of the rural surgical experience has been fully appreciated and utilized. The Spencer Gulf Rural Health School, established several years ago as part of the Commonwealth Government's plans to increase the exposure of medical undergraduates to the rural sector has been an integral component in the implementation of the surgical program and embraces all facets of rural medical undergraduate education.[21] The effect of eager students gaining a taste for postgraduate rural practice has also been well documented. A North American study concluded that participation in a rural preceptorship in the senior medical undergraduate year was a strong predictor in determining the likelihood of a future rural practice.[22]

More effort needs to be undertaken not only to entice surgeons to rural regions, but also to retain them once they are there. While the university departments cannot control significant influencing factors such as schooling facilities and spouse employment, they can provide substantial support in other areas as evidenced by the described models. The time-honored notion of a single individual being available 24 hours a day, 365 days a year is completely unreasonable in terms of safety for the patient and the well-being of the surgeon. It is time that the community accepts that, to maintain a service, a number of individuals are required.

There is no doubt these models can work, do work, and should be further developed to meet the needs of the Australian rural community and appropriately deploy the scarce surgical resources available.

REFERENCES

1. Kierath A, Hamdorf JM, House AK, et al. Developing visiting surgical services for rural and remote Australian communities. Med J Aust 1998;168(9):454–7.
2. Gruen RL, Bailie RS, d'Abbs PH, et al. Improving access to specialist care for remote Aboriginal communities: evaluation of a specialist outreach service. Med J Aust 2001;174(10):507–11.
3. Bruening MH, Maddern GJ. A profile of rural surgeons in Australia. Med J Aust 1998;169(6):324–6.
4. Green A. Ups and downs of rural practice: a surgeon's view. Med J Aust 1999;171(12):625–6.
5. Bintz M, Cogbill T, Bacon J. Rural trauma care: role of the general surgeon. J Trauma 1996;41(3):462–4.
6. Davies P. Problems with training for general practice in rural South Australia. Med J Aust 1991;55(5):145–7.
7. Royle J. Rural surgery initiatives. RACS Bull 1996;16:42.
8. Australian Medical Workforce Advisory Committee. The general surgery workforce in Australia. Sydney NSW: AMWAC; 1997. (AMWA Report 1997.2).
9. Gadiel D, Ridoutt L. The specialist medical workforce and specialist service provision in rural areas. Canberra ACT: AGPS; 1994. (MWDRC Consultancies No.1).
10. Kamien M, Buttfield IH. Some solutions to the shortage of general practitioners in rural Australia. Part 4. Professional, social and economic satisfaction. Med J Aust 1990;153(3):168–71.
11. Faris I. The making of a rural surgeon. Aust N Z J Surg 1997;67(4):153–6.
12. Rural Specialists Group of the Rural Doctors Association of Australia. A sustainable specialist workforce for rural Australia. 2005. Available at: www.rdaa.com.au. Accessed November, 2008.
13. AMA. National Code of Practice—hours of work, shiftwork and rostering for hospital doctors 1999. Available at: www.ama.com.au. Accessed November, 2008.
14. Azer SA, Simmons D, Elliott SL. Rural training and the state of rural health services: effect of rural background on the perception and attitude of first-year medical students at the University of Melbourne. Aust J Rural Health 2001;9(4):178–85.
15. Rolfe IE, Pearson SA, O'Connell DL, et al. Finding solutions to the rural doctor shortage: the roles of selection versus undergraduate medical education at Newcastle. Aust N Z J Med 1995;25(5):512–7.
16. Bruening MH, Maddern GJ. The provision of general surgical services in rural South Australia: a new model for rural surgery. Aust N Z J Surg 1998;68(11):764–8.

17. Bruening MH, Maddern GJ. Surgical undergraduate education in rural Australia. Arch Surg 2002;137(7):794–8.
18. Bruening MH, Maddern GJ. Student attitudes to surgical teaching in provincial hospitals. Aust J Rural Health 2003;11(3):121–3.
19. Culhane A, Kamien M, Ward A. The contribution of the undergraduate rural attachment to the learning of basic practical and emergency procedural skills. Med J Aust 1993;159(7):450–2.
20. Tulloh B, Clifforth S, Miller I. Caseload in rural general surgical practice and implications for training. Aust N Z J Surg 2001;71(14):215–7.
21. Khadra M. Undergraduate rural clinical schools. Aust N Z J Surg 2001;71(Suppl): A83.
22. Rabinowitz HK, Diamond JJ, Markham FW, et al. Critical factors for designing programs to increase the supply and retention of rural primary care physicians. JAMA 2001;286(9):1041–8.

Surgery in Remote and Rural Scotland

Andrew J.W. Sim, MS, FRCS (Glasgow)[a,b,*],
Fiona Grant, RGN, BSc, Dip. N, MBA, MIHM[c],
Annie K. Ingram, BA, LLM, PhD, FCIPD, MIHM[d,e]

KEYWORDS

• Remote • Rural • Surgery • Rural general hospital

More than 90% of Scotland's land mass is classified as rural, and as many as 1 million of the 5.2 million people in Scotland live in rural areas. The average population density of rural Scotland is 21 persons per square kilometer. Some areas, such as the Western Isles, are more sparsely populated (population density, 9). Access to the remote areas can be difficult and nearly half of the rural population have driving times to population centers of 30,000 of more than hour. As many as 100,000 people live on Scotland's 96 inhabited islands (2001 census); the largest island, Lewis and Harris, is home to 20,000, and only two other islands, Mainland Shetland and Mainland Orkney, have populations greater than 10,000. Scheduled travel to and from the islands is by ferry and small plane. Inclement weather can completely isolate island and more remote communities but rarely for longer than 24 hours.

Medical care to patients in remote and rural Scotland is provided by the National Health Service (NHS). The NHS in Scotland is a devolved responsibility of the Scottish Government and little or no private medical care is provided in the remote and rural areas. The Scottish Government is committed to providing as much health care as near to patients' homes as possible. Local health care provision is the responsibility of NHS Boards. Except for the three island health boards (Orkney, Shetland, and the Western Isles), rural areas are covered by health boards that also care for large cities. NHS Highland, based in Inverness, serves a population of 299,000 and covers an area of 32,518 km^2 (12,507 square miles), which is more than 40% of the Scottish

---

[a] Western Isles Hospital, Macaulay Road, Stornoway, Isle of Lewis, HS1 2AF, Scotland, UK
[b] University of the Highlands and Islands Millennium Institute, Ness Walk, Inverness, IV3 5SQ, Scotland, UK
[c] North of Scotland Planning Group (NoSPG), Administration Block, Spynie Hospital, Duffus Road, Elgin IV30 5PW, UK
[d] Remote and Rural Healthcare, UK
[e] Regional Planning & Workforce Development, NoSPG, Ashludie Hospital, Monifeith, Angus DD5 40HQ, UK
* Corresponding author. Western Isles Hospital, Macaulay Road, Stornoway, Isle of Lewis, HS1 2AF, Scotland, UK.
E-mail address: simajw@yahoo.co.uk (A.J.W. Sim).

Surg Clin N Am 89 (2009) 1335–1347
doi:10.1016/j.suc.2009.09.012
0039-6109/09/$ – see front matter © 2009 Elsevier Inc. All rights reserved.
surgical.theclinics.com

land surface and is an area the size of Belgium. In 2007/2008, the NHS budget was £9.5 billion, and across Scotland an average of £1934 was spent on health care per person per year. Underlining the higher cost of island health care, the only purely nonurban health boards, Orkney, Shetland, and the Western Isles, had approximately £500 per person per year more than the national average.

MILESTONES IN THE DEVELOPMENT OF THE RURAL HOSPITAL SURGICAL SERVICE

The traditional view of the rather eccentric single-handed surgeon working long hours to serve people living in the more isolated areas of Scotland is illustrated by a description from 1913:

> Dr Mackenzie of Uist ... had to operate in a hut on a case of strangulated hernia where a clerk gave chloroform and light was obtained from a tallow candle held by a neighbouring crofter who fainted during the proceedings ....[1]

Conditions have since improved, and surgery in rural Scotland is coming of age and is now a defined and robust part of the NHS. This advancement is a result of the sustained efforts of a small group of dedicated people working over the past 10 to 15 years.

Early Days

Sir John Dewar's report[2] of the Highlands and Islands Medical Service Committee in 1912 graphically described the disastrous situation for health care delivery in isolated areas of Scotland in the early years of the 20th century. His recommendations led to the Highlands and Islands (Medical Services) Grant Act 1913, which provided £42,000 for improving medical services, including nursing, and paved the way for the development approximately 36 years later of the NHS in the United Kingdom.

The First Rural Surgeons

By the mid-1920s, trained specialist general surgeons were attached to hospitals in Lerwick (Shetland), Kirkwall (Orkney), Stornoway (Isle of Lewis), and Wick (Caithness). The effect of these appointments was to increase the number of operations performed locally. After the appointment of J. Ewart Purves in 1925 to the Lewis hospital, Stornoway, operations increased from 60 in 1923 to 551 in 1929.[1] Over the next 50 to 60 years, single handed surgeons working in isolated hospitals performed emergency and elective procedures to a standard acceptable to the local populations; procedures such as appendicectomy, peptic ulcer surgery, cholecystectomy, and inguinal hernia repair were commonplace.

Late 20th Century

The 1980s, 1990s, and early years of the new millennium marked the demise of the single-handed surgeon. Locally based surgical services in the small hospitals located in Golspie, Skye, the Isle of Arran, Stranraer, and South Uist were closed and additional surgeons added to the complement in Shetland, Orkney, Wick, Stornoway, Fort William, and Oban.

The Royal College of Surgeons of Edinburgh

A report by the Royal College of Surgeons of Edinburgh in May 1995 (*Surgery in Hospitals Serving Isolated Communities*) highlighted major problems favouring the withdrawal of locally resident consultant surgical care in isolated areas. These shortcomings reflected a professional view, and included the following:

- Population size, which was insufficient to provide a workload necessary for a surgeon to maintain skills.

- The professional isolation, which led surgeons to continue practices that were outdated and unacceptable.
- The continuous on-call commitment of single-handed surgeons.
- The risk that surgeons may undertake procedures without adequate medical, nursing, and technical backup.
- The recognition that patients who have more serious problems can be more effectively treated in specialized centers.
- Higher surgical training was becoming more specialized and the broadly trained surgeon with wide experience was becoming a rarity.
- Surgeons in some communities had shown versatility and expertise but most were in their mid- to late 50s, and replacing them would be problematic.

Notwithstanding this professional view, local populations usually were known to be satisfied with the treatment provided by their small hospitals, and some remote areas are at a real risk for being isolated by bad weather.

In considering these seemingly opposing camps of opinion, the College Working Group allowed pragmatism to reign and made recommendations for areas where resident surgical services should be maintained and also for areas where surgical services should be withdrawn. To maintain locally based surgical services, regions should have at least two consultant surgeons, potential appointees should be identified early in their training and be specifically trained to work in isolated hospitals, strong links with main hospitals must be established, proper transfer arrangements for patients requiring specialist treatment must be in place, at least two consultant anesthetists should be available, adequate laboratory and radiologic services should be present, and video links with a major accident and emergency department and orthopaedic unit should be established.

In July of 1998, a further report by a working party of the Royal College of Surgeons of Edinburgh (Surgery in Isolated Communities) defined the hospital serving an isolated community as:

An existing hospital with its surgical services provided by a locally based resident, as opposed to visiting, Consultant surgical staff. The hospital must be at least one and a half hours by road from the nearest district general hospital and servicing a population of 30,000 or less.[3]

Six hospitals in Scotland met these criteria: the Gilbert Bain Hospital in Lerwick, Shetland; the Balfour Hospital in Kirkwall, Orkney; the Caithness General Hospital in Wick; the Belford hospital in Fort William; the Lorne and Islands Hospital in Oban and the Western Isles Hospital in Stornoway. At that time, 11 surgeons and 12 anaesthetists were working in these hospitals. In 1998, the working party identified plans to increase the number of surgeons at that time to a total of 15 remote rural hospital consultant surgeons, and suggested that one consultant needed to be trained every 2 years. They provided detailed recommendations for the training of surgeons destined to work in hospitals serving isolated communities.

Scottish Executive or Scottish Government Reports

In 1998, the Acute Services Review Report[4] to the Scottish Office Department of Health by the Chief Medical Officer, Professor Sir David Carter, emphasized the seemingly impossible conundrum that for surgical services in rural (consultant-run) hospitals, the status quo was unsustainable but the downgrading to community (general practitioner–run) hospitals was inappropriate or unachievable. The report recognized that "some characteristics of remoteness strongly favour the continued provision of emergency surgical services" and that "emergency care is at the very heart of any consideration of access to acute services."[4] The report recommended an urgent national exercise to identify and satisfy the future staffing needs of remote communities.

In 2000 the Scottish Executive set up the Remote and Rural Area Resource Initiative (RARARI) to help sustain and improve health care services for people living in the remote and rural areas of Scotland by generating ideas and solutions for: education and training of clinicians, improving patient access, establishing managed clinical networks, sustaining and developing primary care, researching remote and rural health care, and applying telemedicine and its applications. RARARI (AJW Sim, FRCS, personal communication, 2003) appointed a Surgical Educational Facilitator who, with the support of the Viking Surgeons, established an ad hoc working group to consider the effect of contemporary issues on remote and rural surgery. The reports conclusions are listed in **Box 1**.

In the first of his two reports to the Scottish Executive, *Future Practice – A Review of the Scottish Medical Workforce*, Professor Sir John Temple,[5] who was an attendee at the ad hoc working group meetings, expressed clear concerns "that the current arrangements for delivering acute services in small remote and rural hospitals cannot be sustained in isolation where the workload is inadequate to sustain clinical skills…".

This concern was further explored in his second report, *Securing Future Practice – Shaping the New Medical Workforce for Scotland*,[6] when he introduced the concept of defining a set of core services for remote and rural hospitals: "core services are those which need to be delivered 24/7/52 and will require the presence of physicians, surgeons and anaesthetists in the remote centre, integrated with an equivalent team from a larger centre which is prepared to share responsibility for acute clinical care."

The publication of *Building a Health Service Fit for the Future: A National Framework for Service Change in the NHS in Scotland*[7] represented a landmark for rural health care services, and closely impacted on development of the rural surgical service.

Box 1
Conclusions of the Viking Surgeons/RARARI ad hoc working group

1. The specialty of remote and rural surgery should be formalised.

2. Dialog between local populations and Health Boards/Trusts about the future of remote and rural surgical services must be opened.

3. The extent and limits of surgical care in remote and rural hospitals should be defined.

4. All remote and rural surgical units should be linked to a tertiary hospital, which should be responsible for providing surgical care to that remote community.

5. Remote and rural surgical units should have a minimum of three locally based consultant remote and rural surgeons.

6. Remote and rural consultant surgeons should only be available when surgical activity is great enough to require their presence.

7. Acute care specialists should cover the service when consultant surgeons are not available.

8. The threshold for transferring patients from remote and rural hospitals to larger centers should be lowered. Adequate transportation should be provided to meet the increased need.

9. Systems of electronic communication between remote and rural surgical units and larger surgical units must be enhanced.

10. The educational and training needs of locum consultant surgeons in remote and rural hospitals must be supported.

The National Framework for Service Change was informed about rural issues through the work of the Rural Access Action Group. A Rural General Hospital (RGH) model was established and, although not defined, it was expected to provide care in the following areas:

- Emergency medical care: triage, diagnosis, resuscitation, and stabilisation; treat where possible, transfer when necessary
- Locally based routine elective care: diagnosis, treatment or transfer, or follow-up
- Care for chronic illness: care of the elderly, stroke and diabetic care, and renal dialysis

Based on these needs, the RGHs will develop an agreed list of core services. This endeavor is the first time the NHS has attempted to define the services a set of hospitals should provide.

In response to Professor Kerr's report, the Scottish Government established the Remote and Rural Steering Group, which reported its recommendations in November 2007. (Note that initially, after Scottish devolution in 1999, the administrative body of the parliament was called the Scottish Executive, and after the election of the Scottish National Party it became the Scottish Government.) These recommendations were formally endorsed by the Cabinet Secretary for Health and Wellbeing in May 2008 and, through the publication of *Delivering for Remote and Rural Healthcare*,[8] became government policy. This seminal document coined a new, functional definition of the RGH:

The RGH undertakes management of acute medical and surgical emergencies and is the emergency center for the community, including the place of safety for mental health emergencies. It is characterised by more advanced levels of diagnostic services than a Community Hospital and will provide a range of outpatient, day-case, inpatient and rehabilitation services.

The positioning of the RGH on the boundary between the extended clinical care team and the secondary care service and its interactions with community hospitals, District General Hospitals, and tertiary services is clearly shown in **Fig. 1**.

This report identifies the core anesthetic and surgical services to be provided in the RGH.

The anesthetic service has two defined roles: (1) provide emergency care, including resuscitation and stabilization, and administer anesthesia for emergency surgery; and (2) administer anesthesia for elective surgery, which will require a level of activity to maintain skills and retain professional interest. This service will be required 24/7.

The surgical service will provide elective outpatient, inpatient, and day case services and a 24-hour emergency service. The core procedures are listed in **Box 2**.

When breast surgery is to be performed within an RGH, it should be concentrated into the workload of one surgeon, and that surgeon should become part of a formal network with either a District General Hospital or a tertiary center. Services that should be provided by visiting consultant surgeons from a larger hospital include ophthalmology, ear nose and throat surgery, urology, gynaecology, and orthopaedics.

Surgical procedures that should not be considered core within the RGH include:

- Surgery on children younger than 5 years (except for those requiring suture of cuts, drainage of abscesses, and foreign body removal when expertise in pediatric anaesthesia is available)
- Neurosurgery (including emergency burr holes)

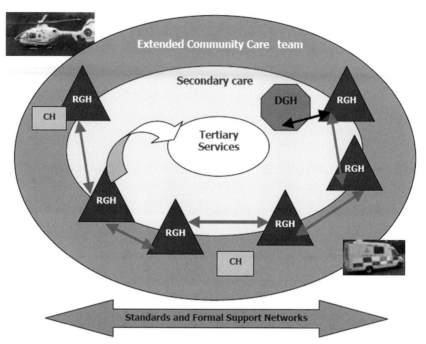

Fig. 1. A diagram of the position of the Rural General Hospital in the proposed schema of health care services for rural populations. CH, community hospital; DGH, District General Hospital; RGH, Rural General Hospital. (*From* NHS Scotland Remote and Rural Steering Group. Delivering for Remote and Rural Healthcare: The Final Report of the Remote and Rural Workstream. Edinburgh: The Scottish Government, 2007; with permission. Crown Copyright © 2008.)

- Operations on the neck and chest (other than emergency tracheostomy)
- Stomach (except perforated and bleeding ulcer surgery) and rectum operations
- Hepatic surgery
- Vascular surgery (other than varicose veins)
- Ovarian surgery (with the exception of cysts with torsion or hemorrhage)
- Vaginal or penile operative procedures (with the exception of circumcision).

When a procedure is needed that is not included within the core list, its performance must be explicitly agreed on through formal governance processes. Approval would be based on demonstration of local health need and team competences, consideration of outcomes expected and approval by the local NHS board.

RGH surgeons should provide outreach day case surgery in community hospitals that have appropriate facilities.

Running parallel to the deliberations of the Remote and Rural Steering Group, a tripartite group, comprising the Academy of Medical Royal Colleges and Faculties in Scotland, NHS Education for Scotland, and the Remote and Rural Steering Group, considered the medical training pathways needed to underpin the delivery of health care to remote and rural patients (the Remote and Rural Training Pathways project). Pathways have been defined for rural general practice, general medicine, general surgery, and anaesthesia.

The final portion of this part of the development of rural surgery is currently being led by the Remote and Rural Implementation Group. This body is tasked by the Scottish

---

Box 2
Core surgical procedures

Emergency surgery

Appendicectomy

Caesarean section

Endoscopy (including injection of varices)

Evacuation of retained products of conception

Exploratory laparotomy

Suture of lacerations

Initial fracture management and joint dislocations

Repair of perforated ulcer

Control of hemorrhage (including splenectomy)

Resection and anastomosis of bowel

Ruptured ectopic pregnancy surgery

Insertion of chest drain

Drainage of pericardium injury (for cardiac tamponade) plus suturing of penetrating injury

Planned surgery

Biopsy of lesions

Cholecystectomy or exploration of common bile duct

Circumcision

Diagnostic cystoscopy

Gastrointestinal endoscopy

Hernia repair

Nail bed procedures

Perianal procedures

Resection and anastomosis of bowel

Simple undescended testes repair

Scrotal surgery including vasectomy

Varicose veins surgery

Government to implement the recommendations of Delivering for Remote and Rural Healthcare[8] across the country.

PRESENT DAY RURAL SURGERY

Patients in the rural areas of Scotland will receive their surgical care locally as much as is feasible. The local surgical care will be provided in a RGH or a community hospital served by visiting surgeons or general practitioners (GPs) who have a special interest in surgery. After referral or consultation, a patient may travel to a larger, usually mainland city hospital for care that cannot be provided closer to home. These transfers are covered by service level agreements.

Specialty surgeons (orthopaedics, urologists, ophthalmologists, otorhinolaryngologists and gynaecologists) travel from larger centers to community hospitals and RGHs to provide outpatient and some operative care. If the rural hospital is outside the area covered by the health board by which the specialty surgeon is normally employed, a service level agreement, which includes details of the financial considerations, is negotiated and agreed. Once the service level agreement is complete, patients move freely between hospitals when clinically necessary. Patient travel is financed centrally by "top slicing" from the Scottish Government's health budget; no personal or health board charging is involved.

Patient Transportation

The Scottish Ambulance Service has prime responsibility for patient transportation. It is run as a nonterrestrial health board for the whole of the country. Road ambulances are plentiful in urban areas but, by necessity, are fewer in rural areas. In rural areas, most ambulances are double-manned with a paramedic and a driver.

The ambulance service has national targets for response times:

- Category A calls: 63% of calls should be responded to within 8 minutes, with this target increasing to 75% by the latter quarter of 2007/2008.
- Category B calls: 95% of category B calls are responded to within 14, 19, or 21 minutes, depending on population density. All rural areas have a 21-minute response target.
- GP urgent calls: 95% of GP calls should have a crew in attendance within 15 minutes of the agreed timescale.

Data from a survey performed for the Remote and Rural Steering Group evaluating ambulance response times in settlements along the most northerly coast of Scotland illustrate the difficulties of meeting national targets, particularly in the more isolated areas, such as Lochninver and Bettyhill (**Table 1**).

The Scottish Ambulance Service provides the air ambulance service. Scotland has two fixed-wing King Air planes and two Eurocopters based in Glasgow, Aberdeen, and Inverness. In times of great need, Coast Guard or Ministry of Defence aircraft (usually helicopters) are mobilized for patient transport.

The first air ambulance flight[9] occurred on May 14, 1933, when John McDermid, who had a perforated duodenal ulcer, was flown from Islay to Renfrew. The first flight to the Outer Hebrides was organized by Dr Alex J Macleod and occurred approximately 8 days later when the Reverend Malcolm Gillies of Clachan Church North Uist, in the terminal stages of his illness, was flown home from Glasgow.

A survey of air ambulance patient transfers in the Western Isles from April 2001 to March 2004 showed an average of one air ambulance transfer to or from the islands per day. Of these, 245 were from the Isle of Barra, 31 by helicopter, and 214 by fixed-wing aircraft (at that time the Islander air ambulance plane was in use and landed

Settlement	Category A (%)	Category B (%)	General Practitioner Urgent Calls (%)
Lochinver	16.7	53.6	97.5
Bettyhill	1.0	76.2	94.3
Thurso	54.6	88.5	97.1
Wick	60.3	89.6	97.3

Table 1
Ability to meet national targets

and took off from the cockle shell beach of Traigh Mhor). Nearly a third (72) of the Barra transfers were emergencies.

The person who accompanies the patient during emergency transportation is determined by the severity of the condition and the availability of staff. Three broad groups of people are available: ambulance paramedics, locally available staff (usually anesthetists), and retrieval teams. Most emergency transfers are safely effected with paramedic staff; medical staff only have a role when the patient is unstable, requires ventilatory support, or requires ongoing resuscitative care. Using a locally based anaesthetic consultant to transfer a severely ill or injured patient from an RGH to a bigger unit causes staff depletion at the rural site and produces the difficulty of returning that staff member to base. No overall national retrieval team service is available in Scotland; only neonatal and paediatric retrieval teams.

A "shock" team based in Glasgow covers the West of the country, and consists of an anaesthetist and specialist nurse who, after consultation between the responsible surgeon and anaesthetist, travel to the Rural General or community hospital by air ambulance. Once there, they assess and stabilize the patient before transfer (usually ventilated) to a mainland intensive care unit. RGHs have high-dependency facilities and can ventilate patients for up to 24 hours, but none has an intensive care unit.

A pilot study is nearing completion of an air ambulance–based Emergency Retrieval Service to transfer severely ill or injured patients from rural areas (including RGHs and community hospitals), with a philosophy more akin to "scoop and run." The objectives of this pilot are to:

- Create an integrated and well governed system of rural emergency care
- Augment rural health care practitioner training in emergency care and transfer
- Provide online expert advice on patient management and transfer
- Provide rapid on-site emergency and critical care interventions
- Safely transfer patients directly to definitive care

The Six Rural General Hospitals

The Scottish Government's publication, *Delivering for Remote and Rural Healthcare: The Final Report of the Remote and Rural Workstream,*[8] formally endorses the existence of the six RGHs and delineates their core activities. The services these hospitals are expected to provide are listed in **Box 3**.

At the time of writing, much of this core activity is available in the six RGHs, and some have additional services. Caithness General Hospital in Wick and the Western Isles Hospital in Stornoway, Isle of Lewis, have consultant-run obstetric and gynaecologic services, and the Western Isles Hospital has a single-handed orthopaedic surgeon consultant who undertakes joint replacement surgery locally.

Surgeons at Rural General Hospitals

Each RGH has at least three consultant surgeons, but not all are permanent employees. As many as 50% are locums consultants, mostly in long-term (>3 months) posts. The General Medical Council requires surgeons to be on the Specialist Register (certifying that they have completed an approved training program) before being appointed to a permanent consultant post. Many surgeons have the skills and experience necessary to work in an RGH but have not yet acquired specialist registration, either through completing an approved training program or having their training and experience evaluated and approved by the Post Graduate Medical Education and Training Board. Until the shortage of trained and registered surgeons for rural areas is resolved, locum surgeons will be employed for both short and long periods.

Box 3
Core services of the six Rural General Hospitals in Scotland

A nurse-led urgent care service to manage minor injury and minor illness, and undertake the initial management of fractures and manipulation of joints.

Ability to resuscitate patients and manage acute surgical and medical admissions; high-dependency care must be available.

Clear and appropriate retrieval and transfer arrangements must be available for patients who cannot be cared for locally.

At a minimum, a midwifery-led maternity service with facility for neonatal resuscitation must be available.

Expertise to diagnosis and initially manage the acutely ill or injured child must be available, and much ambulatory care for children should be possible within the locality.

Management of patients with long-term conditions, including hemodialysis, and cancer care should be available as part of a network with a larger unit; most stroke care should be available locally.

Facilities to continue patient care after major surgery elsewhere should be available.

Routine elective surgery should be performed if included in core procedures list (see **Box 1**).

Visiting services by specialists from larger units are essential and can include ear, nose, and throat surgery; ophthalmology; urology; oncology; orthopaedic surgery; and gynaecology, along with a series of medical and paediatric specialties.

Diagnostic imaging support must be available in the form of routine digitised image capture (for national transmission with the picture archiving and communication system), ultrasound, and CT scanning.

Laboratory services, including a limited range of biochemistry, hematology and blood cross-matching, should be available

Diagnostic and limited therapeutic upper and lower gastrointestinal endoscopy and cystoscopy should be possible.

Cardiac investigation with stress testing and echocardiography should be available.

Pharmaceutical support should be present.

Although the surgical work is similar among RGHs, variations exist that are associated with geographic location and available services. The Belford Hospital in Fort William receives more patients experiencing trauma from climbing and hill-walking injuries sustained in the surrounding hills and mountains (Ben Nevis and the Cairngorms), whereas the surgeons in Orkney and Shetland must perform emergency obstetric procedures (eg, Caesarian section), and the hospitals with active fishing ports see more injuries and conditions associated with fishermen (eg, Injuries from the venomous spine of the ratfish: two case reports and a survey of fishermen; Hayes AJ, MBChB, personal communication, 2009).

The individual surgeon's work is illustrated in the log book the principal author kept while working in the Western Isles Hospital. On average, over the 5-year period from 2004 to 2008, 1200 to 1500 patients were seen in outpatient clinics per year, with 400 to 500 being new referrals. Every year approximately 400 patients were treated as inpatients and 400 as day cases. Between 500 and 600 procedures per year were performed, 300 of which were gastrointestinal endoscopies. Of the operative procedures (approximately 300), 50 to 60 were of moderate or major severity (30–40 cholecystectomies, mainly laparoscopic and 10 to 15 colonic resections, none laparoscopic).

Hospital stays were marginally higher but in-hospital mortality was lower than the national average.

Controversy remains as to whether this workload is sufficient to maintain the skills of rural surgeons. Data from the United States on workload and practice patterns[10] suggest that the number and distribution of procedures is consistent with that undertaken by surgeons applying for reaccreditation. Unlike many urban hospitals in the United Kingdom, where much of the surgical work falls to trainees, the bulk of the surgical work in the RGH is performed by the consultant; because of this, benchmarking the RGH consultants' surgical workload with that of urban hospitals is fraught with difficulty.

Networks with other units exist mainly as personal arrangements and are therefore vulnerable. The future development of obligate networks between rural and larger units, which are underpinned by effective service level agreements, should guarantee a continuing support system for the management of rural surgical patients. Enhanced use of telemedicine and videoconferencing will make use of modern technology for rural surgical care.

An example of effective videoconferencing is the gastrointestinal malignancy multi-disciplinary meeting, which meets weekly (continuously since 2005) by way of video-link. This conference involves surgeons in Caithness General Hospital, Wick, the Belford Hospital in Fort William, and the Western Isles Hospital in Stornoway, linking them to surgeons, physicians, histopathologists, radiologists, and oncologists in the District General Hospital, Raigmore, in Inverness. The clinical details, histopathology, and radiologic images are available for all to see, and an individual management plan is decided for all patients who have gastrointestinal malignancy.

Surgical Education and Training in Rural General Hospitals

Undergraduate

Most if not all of the surgical units in Scotland's RGHs host periods of study for undergraduate medical students. Many are final-year students from the University of Aberdeen, but others come from other Scottish and United Kingdom Universities or European Union and Commonwealth Universities. In general terms, these study periods are underpinned by three objectives:

1. To provide a general, broad-based period of study in an environment where the care pathway of a patient can be witnessed from beginning to end.
2. To show how patients in a rural environment are managed and how a more holistic and patient-centered health system is available away from urban centers.
3. To showcase rural surgery and present it as a positive career option.

A study of undergraduate attitudes toward placement in a rural environment, determined through an undergraduate assessment of the impact on medical training of a remote and rural clinical attachment, which was presented at the Making it Work 2 program[11] in 2005, showed that the broad range of skills required for rural practice appealed to most (91%), and that 79% would be interested in a specific training program if available. This study showed that undergraduates experienced more educational opportunities and had more general clinical, hands-on, and practical experience in the rural hospital than in any of their previous clinical placements. Of the 35 undergraduates surveyed, 29 believed they would be more likely to work in a remote community because of their experience.

Postgraduate (generic)

The newly introduced nationwide compulsory Foundation Program has allowed more newly qualified doctors to experience rural practice than ever before. More than

20 doctors per year in the North of Scotland Deanery's program will experience rural general hospital surgery in either the first or second year of their professional lives. For many years, the Western Isles Hospital has had a trainee from the South East Scotland surgical training program.

Postgraduate (specific)

The Remote and Rural Training Pathways project proposed the construction of a curriculum for remote and rural surgical practice from the Intercollegiate Surgical Curriculum project and the Orthopaedic Competence Assessment project. This curriculum would include abstraction of the knowledge base and necessary competences required of a surgeon working in relative isolation. Furthermore, the project suggested that

> Surgeons in remote and rural practice require a broad generic training and that this would include experience in some aspects of emergency medicine (formerly Accident and Emergency (A&E)), orthopaedic surgery, urology, obstetrics and gynaecology, neurosurgery, otorhinolaryngology, ophthalmology and plastic surgery. Most of these elements could be achieved during attachment to busy A&E Departments with secondments to specialist departments built into the curriculum. In some specialties, neurosurgery for example, the trainee would be required to acquire understanding of the principles of the specialty rather than a list of specific skills since there would be very few occasions in which these skills would be required.[7]

The North of Scotland Deanery has a program specifically designed to produce RGH surgeons. This training includes the recommendations of the Remote and Rural Training Pathway project and provides the opportunity to work in one or more of the RGHs. Two trainees are nearing completion of this specialist training program and should be eligible to apply for consultant posts within the next 2 or 3 years. Posts are also available for trainees nearing the completion of their specialist general surgical training to embark on a specific 2-year rural training as a part of a rural surgical fellowship program; 1 individual is in-post.

Ad hoc rural training posts exist elsewhere in the country and one individual is undertaking rural surgical training in Northern Ireland. Ideally, appointments would be made to RGHs in a proleptic manner and would allow directed surgical training; however, United Kingdom regulations currently do not permit this for any period greater than the 6 months before obtaining the certificate of completion of specialist training. Only one of the RGH consultant surgeons in-post has undergone specific rural surgical training.

The Viking Surgeons Group

In 1973, a group of single-handed surgeons working in isolated hospitals in Scotland and other parts of the United Kingdom met in Stornoway and formed the Viking Surgeons Group. The group shares experiences, invites speakers to deliver updates on relevant advances in surgery, and learns about specific practices in the host's area of practice. The Viking Surgeons have met every year for the past 36 years; whenever possible, the meetings have been hosted alternately on a mainland or island location. Partners (usually wives) attend and a specific program is organized for them.

The format of the meeting has been established and comprises a day of lectures and presentations, an annual general meeting, and a formal dinner at which the Viking lecture is delivered. The two Viking helmets are passed on from the previous meeting's organizer to the present meeting's organizer at the dinner. The second day features lectures in the morning and a cultural visit in the afternoon. A golf competition for the Viking Shield is held on the day before the meeting.

It is considered an honor to be asked to make a presentation to the Viking Surgeons. Over the years, members have come from the isolated hospitals in Scotland, Penzance in England, the Isle of Man, the Faroe Islands, and Iceland. Meetings in the past few years have been held in Iceland, Shetland, Oban, Orkney, Wick, Stornoway, Fort William, Northern Ireland, and Elgin. At the 2002 meeting in Oban, the Viking Surgeons decided to look into contemporary issues affecting the practice of rural surgery. They were specifically tasked to study Professor Sir John Temple's report,[5] the New Consultant's Contract, and the European Working Time Regulations, marking the first time the Viking Surgeons entered the medicopolitical arena. As the only body representing views of practicing rural hospital doctors, their view was much sought after and the dialog that occurred in the Ad Hoc Working Group meetings formed the basis for future deliberations about rural surgery in Scotland.

CONCLUSION

Over the past 15 years, rural surgery in Scotland has emerged from the backwaters of the Scottish Health service to a recognized and important part of overall health care provision in Scotland. No longer is the rural surgeon regarded by his city colleague as the eccentric poor relation of the urban specialist. The rural surgeon is now more likely to have the skills and experience necessary for the work that must be done. Training pathways are defined to ensure succession planning. The support of the Scottish Government, Health Boards, and the Royal Colleges has been essential; their continued involvement will ensure safe surgery for those who dwell in the more isolated areas of Scotland.

REFERENCES

1. Crosfill M. The Highlands and Islands Medical Service: precursor of a state funded medical care system. Vesalius 1996;2(2):118–25.
2. The Highlands and Islands Medical Service Committee. Report to the Lords Commissioners of His Majesty's Treasury (The Dewar Report). Edinburgh, Scotland: HMSO; 1912.
3. Working Party Report: Surgery in isolated communities, Royal College of Surgeons of Edinburgh, 1998.
4. Acute services review. Scottish Office Department of Health. Edinburgh: Scottish Office Publications; 1998. Available at: www.scotland.gov.uk/deleted/library/document5/acute-00.htm.
5. Temple JG. Future practice: a review of the Scottish medical workforce. Edinburgh, Scotland: Scottish Executive Health Department; 2002.
6. Temple JG. Securing future practice shaping the new medical workforce for Scotland. Edinburgh, Scotland: Scottish Executive Health Department; 2004.
7. Building a health service fit for the future: a national framework for service change in the NHS in Scotland. Edinburgh, Scotland: Scottish Executive; 2005.
8. Delivering for remote and rural healthcare: the final report of the remote and rural workstream. Edinburgh, Scotland: The Scottish Government; 2008. p. 70.
9. Hutchison I. Jimmy and the dragon. In: Air Ambulance - Six decades of the Scottish Air Ambulance Service. Scotland, United Kingdom: Kea Publishing; 1996. p. 11–5.
10. Ritchie WP Jr, Rhodes RS, Biester TW. Work loads and practice patterns of general surgeons in the United States, 1995–1997: a report from the American Board of Surgery. Ann Surg 1999;230(4):533–42.
11. Making It Work 2 Conference. Tromsø, Norway, September 21–22, 2005. Abstract Book. p. 17–8. Available at: http://www.helsenord.no/getfile.php/RHF/Prosjekter/Making%20it%20Work/Abstract_book_Making_it_Work2_2005.pdf.

Building and Maintaining a Successful Surgery Program in Rural Minnesota

Howard M. McCollister, MD[a,b,*], Paul A. Severson, MD[a,b],
Timothy P. LeMieur, MD[c], Shawn A. Roberts, MD[c],
Mark W. Gujer, MD[d]

KEYWORDS

• MIMIS • Cuyuna • Rural • MIS • Minnesota • NSQIP

For decades, it has been axiomatic that rural health care systems are crucial factors not only in the health of the populations that they serve but also in the viability of America's rural communities. Medical care, as it is delivered in rural America, is becoming increasingly problematic as national health care delivery models continue to evolve. Increasing reimbursement pressures and changing practitioner lifestyle expectations had a variety of negative effects on the health of rural communities and the populations they serve. The results of those pressures have consistently and repeatedly been manifested across the country by rural hospital closings[1] and a declining level of surgical care available. These two factors are interrelated, given the importance of surgical services to the revenue stream of any hospital.

Our involvement with rural surgery programs—our own, at two rural critical access hospitals (CAHs); our regional rural surgery service consulting work; statewide conferences; and national venues, such as the semiannual Rural Surgery Symposium sponsored by the Mithoefer Center for Rural Surgery[2]—has led us to the conclusion that the basic model for rural surgery practice in America is in serious

[a] Minnesota Institute for Minimally Invasive Surgery, Cuyuna Regional Medical Center, 318 East Main Street, Crosby, MN 56441, USA
[b] Bariatric Surgery Division, Minnesota Institute for Minimally Invasive Surgery, Cuyuna Regional Medical Center, Crosby, 318 East Main Street, Crosby, MN 56441, USA
[c] Minnesota Institute for Minimally Invasive Surgery, Cuyuna Regional Medical Center, 318 East Main Street, Crosby, MN 56441, USA
[d] Department of Anesthesia, Minnesota Institute for Minimally Invasive Surgery, Crosby, MN, USA
* Corresponding author. Minnesota Institute for Minimally Invasive Surgery, Cuyuna Regional Medical Center, 318 East Main Street, Crosby, MN 56441.
E-mail address: hmccollister@clmc.sisunet.org (H.M. McCollister).

Surg Clin N Am 89 (2009) 1349–1357
doi:10.1016/j.suc.2009.09.011
0039-6109/09/$ – see front matter © 2009 Elsevier Inc. All rights reserved.

jeopardy as reimbursement and provider models evolve. The conventional rural surgery model of providing hernia/gallbladder surgery, basic trauma, cesarean sections, and basic gynecologic and orthopedic surgery is going to have limited and decreasing sustainability in the coming years. This has been troubling as we see these things representing the basic thrust of this country's nascent rural surgery postgraduate training programs. They must be a vital component of such training, but by themselves, they represent rural surgical programs that are ultimately doomed to failure as a broad-based solution to the surgical needs of the rural populations and the viability of the health care institutions that those programs need to serve. These conventional programs may serve to meet current local needs, but they emphasize breadth of services rather than depth, and, without the background or resources available to provide modern, advanced surgical services, their ability to grow and compete is impaired. Their growth becomes dependent entirely on the growth of their local populations rather than providing a viable alternative to larger nearby institutions.

Our experience has been that a rural surgery program does have to be broadly based in the service it provides but to sustain its growth, it must be surgeon directed and centered on modern surgical practice. In today's surgical world, that means flexible endoscopy, minimally invasive surgery (MIS), and advanced laparoscopic techniques. As those techniques continue to evolve, all surgical practices—rural and urban—must evolve with them or risk being left behind. If they are left behind, they will die, no matter how many hernia/gallbladder operations or cesarean sections are performed. In that regard, the importance of flexible endoscopy, including screening programs (colon and Barrett's esophagus), and flexible endosurgery cannot be overemphasized. In addition to providing direct revenue, these procedures serve as springboards to the identification of a wide variety of gastrointestinal disease, wherein surgical treatment represents an appropriate solution and those operations are preserved for the local system. This in turn requires that a surgery department be capable of addressing them using modern surgical techniques. It does little good for a system if a local surgeon-endoscopist identifies intractable gastroesophageal reflux disease yet is unable to perform a laparoscopic Nissen fundoplication or identifies a colon cancer but cannot offer a laparoscopic colon resection. A scenario even more problematic for a local system is one where all flexible endoscopy is referred to remote gastroenterologists. Patients are generally more likely to get their operation, if indeed such an operation is deemed necessary by a gastroenterologist, within that medical specialist's own referral system.

COMPONENTS OF A SUCCESSFUL RURAL SURGERY PROGRAM

There are many components to a successful surgery program, rural or urban, and the extent to which these components are identified and implemented is directly related to the extent of that success. These components go beyond doing competent surgery and extend into areas of education and leadership. Educational programs for the public enhance information, visibility, and community pride as the programs generate awareness of various disease topics and what advanced surgical options are available to them locally. Educational seminars are no less important for a surgery program's local referral primary care base, for largely the same reasons. The extent to which such educational opportunities can be extended to regional primary health care providers has the added benefit of expanding a program's referral base, just as regional informational patient education seminars can expand a surgical patient base beyond the local area.

If a surgical practice is successful in establishing a level of expertise in a given area, we have found that it is important to do whatever is possible to share that expertise with surgical colleagues in surrounding areas. This may seem counterintuitive to the extent that it provides competing practices with equal expertise, but it has been apparent to us that it is generally more detrimental to have these operations done poorly by regional colleagues, as subsequent word-of-mouth may convince patients that they should go outside the region for their care.

Participation in educational programs for medical students (on-site lecturing or in-house preceptorships) is another way to promote a medical system, which in turn may pay dividends down the road when recruiting new doctors for a system. Likewise, it can be useful to provide educational opportunities to residents in training programs. These young doctors, if they are not ultimately recruited to a medical system, may well end up being colleagues (and potential referral sources) in surrounding areas.

One of the most important, and most obvious, components of a successful surgery program is a successful primary care program. As a referral gateway, competent and accessible primary care doctors are vital, and it is important that a surgery program be involved in the design and recruiting of that component of the medical system.

Although it runs counter to the traditional concepts of what a rural surgeon is and does and what rural medical programs are and should be, it is our contention that the rural medical systems that have a surgery program, or are recruiting one, must be prepared to grow beyond the classic rural surgery model in order be viable into the future. Solo surgeons trying to cover the surgical needs of a rural medical system by themselves are going to face the issues that have placed rural surgery programs in trouble in the first place: professional isolation and stressful lifestyle. As the lifestyle expectations of today's generation of physicians permeate the medical and surgical workforce, the likelihood that those issues will be impediments to recruitment and retention of rural surgeons likewise increases. The logical progression of that concept is that a rural surgery practice must be able to evolve beyond the all-rural surgery performed by a general surgeon with the goal that it becomes feasible to recruit not only a general surgery partner but also other core surgical specialties. Adding, over time, obstetrician/gynecologists, orthopedists, and anesthesiologists can exponentially increase the breadth of surgical services a system can provide, thereby also increasing revenue for the rural health care system. In our opinion, this is the progression of success: a single rural general surgeon expands services and gets busy enough to recruit a partner; that practice gets busy enough doing basic orthopedics and gynecology to recruit specialists in those areas, in turn creating a need for a broadly capable anesthesia program in these heavily Medicare-populated areas. Anesthesiologists, in particular, can bring a wide variety of value-added services to a rural system that go beyond adding the ability to do more highly advanced surgical procedures on sicker patients. They can bring expertise to an ICU, streamline the perioperative process, and add important and lucrative services to a system, such as chronic pain management. The addition of these surgical specialties will almost always begin with a viable general surgery program with an aggressive and enterprising rural-trained general surgeon. We believe that if that program does not go on to provide increasing specialty breadth and depth, it will not be sustainable.

Needless to say, such a stepwise growth can be a long and expensive process, requiring the whole-hearted support of an entire medical staff, administration, and hospital trustees. It would be easy for a rural hospital system to breathe a sigh of relief once a rural surgeon is recruited; however, it cannot stop there. The status quo is always easier, but the status quo has a tendency to slide backwards, and this has never been more likely than it is in today's US health care delivery system.

HISTORY OF CUYUNA REGIONAL MEDICAL CENTER

Cuyuna Regional Medical Center (CRMC) is a 25-bed CAH[3] in Crosby, Minnesota (population 2243), and is the parent organization of the Minnesota Institute for Minimally Invasive Surgery (MIMIS). Its four, local, private-practice general surgeons also provide surgical coverage at another nearby CAH, Riverwood Health Care Center, in Aitkin, Minnesota (population 1948). Both of these institutions began in the pre–World War II era in the vein of classic rural medicine, with a general practitioner. The need for enhanced surgical coverage at these two hospitals was clear even then, and those local doctors were ultimately successful in recruiting a university-trained, board-certified general surgeon as he separated from the US Navy Medical Corps in the postwar period. Surgical volume began to build slowly, and the financial benefits of a rural surgery program became increasingly clear to the administrations and hospital boards of these two institutions. Even so, surgical growth in this conventional rural surgery practice was slow. The variety of operations available from this surgeon was in the nature of classic rural surgery—basic orthopedics, gynecology, and general surgery—but the surgical practice offered little by way of breadth of surgical services that might set it apart from a nearby competing surgical practice and provide a competitive advantage. The growth of the surgical practice was thus limited, for the most part, by the slow, or nonexistent, growth of the population of these two small communities.

As this surgical practice languished over the next 3 decades, stable but with little growth, the single surgeon-lynchpin of the system began to face retirement. In 1984, he recruited a young surgeon to replace him. Just out of training, he brought with him a broad range of modern surgical skills but, more importantly, a vision of where such a surgical practice could go. With the aid and teaching of his senior partner, he carried on the traditional rural surgeon's role in basic orthopedics, gynecology, and emergency obstetrics, but more importantly he was also successful in implementing several new programs and a broader range of surgical services. This included a full and flexible endoscopy suite and a modern colonoscopy screening program. The financial benefits to the hospital of these expanded capabilities were immediately recognized and, further, such growth became a priority of the institution. Shortly after the original surgeon at CRMC retired, his young protégé was successful in recruiting a like-minded partner, in 1987. These two young surgeons provided the usual range of rural surgery—hernia and gallbladder, basic orthopedics, gynecologic, and emergency obstetric—and expanded the repertoire of capabilities into the realms of vascular surgery, noncardiac thoracic surgery, and a full range of flexible endoscopy. The system saw substantial growth over the next 3 years. As 1990 ushered in the era of laparoscopic surgery, these two surgeons grasped the significance of the concept and the role it would play in the future of surgery. The entire direction of the practice changed. They became true believers and early adopters of MIS. As new tools and techniques were developed, they were embraced and implemented. In order to help the public become aware of the benefits of MIS, they implemented a variety of community education programs on the topic and its various applications and benefits.

The MIS program began in the typical fashion for MIS programs of the late 1980's—cholecystectomy and pelviscopy—but as the only facility in the region with laparoscopic capability, success began to build rapidly. Dedication to MIS took us into other advanced techniques, including video-assisted thoracoscopic surgery for chest surgery and laparoscopically assisted vaginal hysterectomy. In conjunction with major industry device manufacturers and their sales networks, we were able to establish on-site teaching courses for regional surgeons wishing to learn these advanced techniques. We earned a regional reputation as leaders in advanced laparoscopic surgery and were sought after not only for these courses taught at our institution but also for onsite proctoring and credentialing verification at other surgeons' home hospitals. Our ongoing development of MIS and the associated public education seminars we offered led to a broad-based public reputation for surgical excellence and resultant increased local market penetration. As surgical volumes grew, we found ourselves busy to the point where a third general surgeon was necessary to accommodate that increased volume. That addition was accomplished in 1998. We had gone from a single operating room in 1987 to six operating rooms in 2001, four of which were fully outfitted as complete, endosuites. The ongoing success of CRMC as a thriving rural health care system, as defined by increased surgical volume and revenue, was achieving significant recognition throughout the region and led to consulting agreements at some surrounding hospitals. These consulting programs were designed toward taking those small rural hospitals from surgical programs consisting of surgery performed by local family practitioners and occasional itinerant general surgeons to recruitment of in-house general surgeons performing advanced laparoscopic surgery and flexible endoscopy. The first of these was a 2-year program consisting of 1-day-a-week proctoring of the new local surgeon and teaching him advanced MIS in his own hospital on his own patients. It was successful in generating substantially increased surgical revenue. At the same time, we were developing and implementing teaching programs for other regional surgeons in those same techniques at our own facility and providing 1-month rotations in flexible endoscopy for residents in regional family practice residency programs. Surgical volume and revenue continued to grow, and in 2004 we recruited a fourth general surgeon to our practice as we expanded our foregut surgery program into bariatric surgery.

During the period of expansion into advanced MIS, we continued to provide typical rural surgical services: basic orthopedics, emergency obstetrics, and laparoscopic gynecology. Although we had begun as classic rural surgeons, it had become clear that our medical system could not sustain further growth without moving forward with a broader range of specialty surgery. An important component of this growth strategy was our concept of growing the total surgery program rather than engaging in "turf protection" for the general surgeons. In 2002, we were able to recruit an orthopedic surgeon who was able to take the facility from basic trauma orthopedics to a successful full-spectrum general orthopedic and total joint replacement program. In 2004, we were able to recruit additional orthopedic surgeons, giving us a fellowship-trained joint specialist and a fellowship-trained sports medicine specialist. Gynecologic surgery had been an important portion of our practice, but it was clear that the expanded capabilities brought to the surgery program by two fully trained gynecologists would be beneficial to the overall growth of the facility, and in 2004 we were able to add two obstetrician/gynecologists who had been fully trained in minimally invasive gynecology. Although these specialty additions did initially pull some caseload away from general surgery, it allowed us to concentrate on moving forward with other advanced techniques, such as laparoscopic bariatric surgery and a complete laparoscopic foregut surgery program. It also provided the time necessary to expand our teaching programs and minifellowships for regional surgeons, and we began taking active leadership roles in state, regional, and even national committees and organizations. We were able to thus enhance our regional reputation by establishing a leadership position in a variety of MIS areas.

In 2003, through our participation in state and national surgical organizations, we were encouraged by The Fellowship Council to develop a 1-year fully accredited fellowship program in MIS. After 3 years of development, this fellowship program was provisionally accredited in 2006 and received a full 3-year accreditation in 2007 in the areas of MIS, bariatric surgery, and flexible endosurgery.

Thus, we were able to achieve significant success for the facility's surgery program by growing beyond the traditional role of the rural surgeon and developing a broad-spectrum surgery program in a rural hospital. The distinction between these two concepts is an important one. It has become clear to us that growth is a crucial component of ongoing success and, in this day of expanding surgical tools, techniques, and concepts, that growth entails a broader range of services that these rural hospitals must provide to compete successfully. By sacrificing some of our rural surgery "turf" to more broadly trained specialists, this 25-bed CAH was able to grow beyond classic rural surgery capabilities, and the success of the total program enhanced the success of the individual specialties.

MINNESOTA INSTITUTE FOR MINIMALLY INVASIVE SURGERY

In 2001, CRMC created MIMIS. This was conceived as "brand identification", with commitment to the basic concepts that had led CRMC to the success of its surgery program:

- Surgical excellence—tools and training necessary to perform surgery with quality on par with or better than national standards and outcomes
- Broad capability in advanced MIS surgical techniques—ongoing identification and implementation of new and developing MIS surgical techniques in orthopedics, gynecology, and general surgery
- Education—training of other physicians in endoscopy and advanced MIS techniques. (MIS fellowship, endoscopy training for family practice, and rural surgery rotation for residents at the University of North Dakota)
- Participation in state and national organizations—a seat at the table with well-recognized institutions, such as the University of Minnesota and the Mayo Clinic, and national organizations, such as the American College of Surgeons (ACS) and the Society for American Gastrointestinal and Endoscopic Surgeons (SAGES).

MINNESOTA INSTITUTE FOR MINIMALLY INVASIVE SURGERY TODAY

MIMIS represents all of the in-house surgery programs at CRMC. It consists of 12 surgeons in the specialty areas of general surgery, gynecology, orthopedics, and ophthalmology. We have come to believe strongly that in order for any general surgery program to survive, it must keep abreast of the evolution of general surgery and incorporate MIS as a key component. That applies to rural surgery programs just as it does to urban programs. We have endeavored to follow the concepts with which MIMIS was conceived.

Surgical Excellence

The four laparoendoscopic surgeons work closely and cooperatively. We view our patients as the patients of all of us and collaborate closely on the care of every single one. We have an active and comprehensive quality assurance program that revolves around the National Surgical Quality Improvement Program (NSQIP).[4] This is a comprehensive and predictive national program offered by the ACS for the purpose of measuring and reporting surgical quality and outcomes in a risk-adjusted fashion. By using this database, we are able to constantly compare our surgical outcomes to all other NSQIP facilities across the nation. In 2006 we were also one of 12 centers nationwide invited to participate in the ACS pilot program for extending the NSQIP database to bariatric surgery.

From a patient perspective, we participate in ongoing patient surveys using Press Ganey[5] standardized patient surveys from every single surgical patient coming through our program. In addition, MIMIS and CRMC have sought program accreditation through as many venues as is practical. CRMC, as a facility, is accredited by the Joint Commission.[6] The MIMIS bariatric program and Dr Howard McCollister are accredited by the American Society for Metabolic and Bariatric Surgery center of excellence program,[7] the ACS Bariatric Surgery Center Network,[8] and the Blue Cross/Blue Shield Blue Distinction Center for Bariatric Surgery.[9] We are currently in the process of moving toward establishment of the Greeley hospital accreditation, performance improvement, and safety program.[10]

Broad Capability in Advanced Minimally Invasive Surgery Techniques

We pursue the evaluation and implementation of a wide variety of surgical tools and techniques. We are and have been recruited by several different device manufacturers for the purpose of prototype evaluation and development. We currently offer expertise in a variety of MIS operations in the areas of thoracoscopy, foregut surgery, colon surgery, and solid organ surgery. As a regional referral facility, we have developed extensive experience in reoperative and revisional MIS surgery. Our fully accredited bariatric surgery program offers laparoscopic roux-en-Y, Lap Band, and sleeve gastrectomy operations, and over the 9 years of its existence has never had a patient death. We offer several different flexible endoscopic surgical techniques, including the Stretta procedure, BARRX Halo[360] ablation of Barrett's esophagus, and esophyx transoral intragastric fundoplication. We maintain our own gastrointestinal diagnostics laboratory, including esophageal impedance pH and manometry testing, Bravo wireless ambulatory pH testing, and capsule endoscopy evaluation using PillCam ESO and PillCam SB.

Education

Education has been a key component of our surgery program for decades in several forms. We began by participating in the education of medical students by lecture and as proctors in gross anatomy basic science. We also provide the basic primary surgery clerkship for two medical students per year in their third year as part of the University of Minnesota's Rural Physician Associate Program.[11] Two different family practice residency programs have sought us out to provide a 1-month rotation in flexible endoscopy for second- and third-year residents. We have trained several of these residents who were going to remote rural practices where there was no surgeon available to provide flexible endoscopy services. We have also provided this training and the associated credentialing support to regional surgeons who had never trained in these procedures.

As our expertise in advanced MIS techniques grew, we developed 2-day training programs for surgeons in such procedures as laparoscopic preperitoneal Burch bladder neck suspension, laparoscopic Nissen fundoplication, Trivex varicose vein surgery, and the Ethicon procedure for prolapse and hemorrhoids, stapled hemorrhoidopexy. We have also provided minifellowships in bariatric surgical techniques and with all of these procedures have offered on-site proctoring for these surgeons in their home hospital to achieve the American Medical Association level 4 CME certification required by some hospitals for credentialing. To date, we have trained more than 60 surgeons from four states these techniques.

Education—Minnesota Institute for Minimally Invasive Surgery Fellowship

As we observed the movement of MIS toward becoming the de facto standard for modern surgical technique, we became dismayed at the state of MIS training of many or most of the general surgery residents finishing their residency. We noted that the 87 US fellowships in MIS were becoming the most highly sought-after post-residency training positions offered in the United States. We were also becoming aware, through the Mithoefer Center for Rural Surgery and their semiannual Rural Surgery Symposium, of the looming crisis in rural surgery manpower distribution. We were encouraged by Dr C. Dan Smith, president of The Fellowship Council,[12] to consider establishing such a MIS fellowship at our institution. After 3 years of investigation and preparation, we applied for and received provisional accreditation for our own fellowship in MIS in 2006. We entered our program into the required National Intern and Resident Matching Program match and after interviewing several candidates were fortunate in matching our first choice. During that first year, we were required to apply for full accreditation, and after the on-site review and interview process, we were successful in gaining a full 3-year accreditation in MIS, bariatric surgery, and flexible endosurgery. To date, we are the only accredited fellowship based in a rural CAH, and the only accredited fellowship in the United States or Canada that is able to certify training in all three of those areas. In our second and third years, we were again able to secure our first choices through the match. We have found the program successful and gratifying. Both of the fellows that have finished our program to date have taken their skills to rural America, one of our key goals for this training program.

Participation in State and National Organizations

We believe, in this day of increasing third-party intrusion into health care delivery and decision-making, that it is important to try to develop a high profile among regional, state, and national thought leaders in medicine and surgery. Current and future pressures on cost containment and toward health care reform, or health insurance reform, as the push is now known, have the distinct potential to be detrimental to rural surgical delivery models and their ability to evolve, sustain, and grow a rural surgery program like MIMIS. Consequently we have worked hard to stay involved in regional, state, and national organizations. Some of the four general surgeons are or have been intimately involved in several such groups. The resultant relationships have been important in establishing and maintaining credibility as a surgical program, not just as a rural surgery program. We have been officers, directors, or even founders of all of the surgical societies in this state and have been invited to participate at various committee levels at SAGES and the ACS. The result has been the opportunity to have input into many of the issues that we face every day.

SUMMARY

MIMIS at CRMC in Crosby, Minnesota, is an example of the potential evolution of a successful rural surgical system. In its 24-year history, the facility has gone from one surgeon in the classic rural surgical model to 12 in-house surgeons routinely performing highly advanced surgical procedures in the specialties of general surgery, gynecology, orthopedics, and ophthalmology. This progression has had tremendous financial benefit to this small, rural hospital system and the local community. Our experience and involvement with several other rural medical systems in our region have convinced us that a strong and growing surgical program is essential to the ongoing survivability of these hospital systems that are serving the 23% of Americans who live in our rural communities. To accomplish that growth, rural surgeons and rural surgery training programs much reach beyond the classic model of rural surgery that has been the historical norm for many decades and be certain that they are teaching and applying modern surgical technique in the services they provide. To do otherwise will impair their ability to compete with larger regional facilities and hamper their ability to recruit additional surgeons. The consequence of these problems is lack of growth and failure of the surgery program with loss of the financial benefit that that implies for that rural health care system.

REFERENCES

1. Rehnquist J. Trends in rural hospital closure 1990–2000. OEI 04-02-00610. Washington, DC: US Department of Health and Human Services, Office of Inspector General; 2003.
2. Mithoefer Center for Rural Surgery. Available at: http://www.centerforruralsurgery.org/. Accessed September 18, 2009.
3. Critical Access Hospital. Available at: http://www.doh.wa.gov/hsqa/ocrh/CAH/cah399.html. Accessed September 18, 2009.
4. National Surgical Quality Improvement Program (NSQIP). Available at: http://www.acsnsqip.org/main/about_overview.asp. Accessed September 18, 2009.
5. Press Ganey Associates. Available at: http://www.pressganey.com/cs/our_services. Accessed September 18, 2009.
6. Joint Commission. Available at: http://www.jointcommission.org/. Accessed September 18, 2009.
7. Surgical Review Corporation Center of Excellence Program. Available at: http://www.surgicalreview.org/. Accessed September 18, 2009.
8. American College of Surgeons Bariatric Surgery Centers Network. Available at: http://www.acsbscn.org/Public/index.aspx. Accessed September 18, 2009.
9. Blue Distinction Centers for Bariatric Surgery. Available at: http://www.bcbs.com/innovations/bluedistinction/blue-distinction-bariatric/. Accessed September 18, 2009.
10. Greeley Hospital Accreditation. Performance improvement, and safety program. Available at: http://www.greeley.com/consulting.cfm. Accessed September 18, 2009.
11. University of Minnesota Rural Physician Associate Program (RPAP). Available at: http://www.med.umn.edu/RPAP/. Accessed September 18, 2009.
12. The Fellowship Council. Available at: http://www.fellowshipcouncil.org/. Accessed September 18, 2009.

Rural Surgical Practice: An Iowa Group Model

Timothy A. Breon, MS, MD, FACS

- Rural • Surgery • Practice • Group • Career

The practice of general surgery in rural areas has been studied frequently over the last decade or more.[1–3] An aging population of general surgeons practicing in rural areas combined with fewer young surgeons adequately trained, or even desiring to practice in rural areas, is cause for alarm among many small rural communities.[3,4] Policy-makers are also concerned about retention of surgical services in rural areas because they recognize general surgeons play a vital role in the delivery of health care in rural communities.[5] Although the workforce has been well characterized recently, few recommendations have been offered to help make the practice of general surgery in rural areas more attractive.

Factors that make a career in rural surgery attractive, for some, include living and serving in a small rural and oftentimes underserved community, independence, wide variety of cases, varied employment opportunities, potential for excellent financial rewards, and a happy spouse and family.[5,6] Unfortunately, for others, these same factors can be quite unattractive when considering a location to live and practice surgery. Some of the most significant concerns for surgeons practicing alone in rural areas include being on call continuously and the inability to take vacation or CME leave.

This article describes how Iowa Rural Surgical Associates (IRSA), a group practice, was developed to meet the surgical needs of three rural communities in southeast Iowa. The steps that IRSA has taken developing their group have resulted in a system of surgical delivery that not only improves care but also retains the attractive factors of living and practicing in a rural community. It is hoped that these steps are also helpful to other surgeons.

THE PROBLEM

Iowa is one of the nation's most rural states with 56% of the residents in 88 of 99 counties living outside of metropolitan statistical areas versus only 27% of Americans in the United States living outside of a metropolitan statistical area (county or group of counties with 50,000 or more residents). The patient-to-physician ratio in Iowa

Department of Surgery, Mahaska Health Partnership, Mahaska Health General Surgeons, 410 North 12th Street, Suite 200, Oskaloosa, IA 52577, USA
E-mail address: tbreonmd@irsapc.com

Surg Clin N Am 89 (2009) 1359–1366
doi:10.1016/j.suc.2009.07.012   surgical.theclinics.com
0039-6109/09/$ – see front matter © 2009 Elsevier Inc. All rights reserved.

exceeds 3000:1 in nearly one quarter of rural counties compared with 448:1 among urban citizens and 1639:1 in counties with less than 25,000 persons in the United States of America in 1988.[7] Among the states, Iowa ranks 28th in population, but ranks 38th in certified general surgeons per 100,000 population at 6.06/100,000.[3,4] The surgeon to population ratio in the area served by the surgery practice was 2.5 to 3.75 per 100,000 before the establishment of IRSA. Now, the rate is similar to the statewide average at 6.25 per 100,000.

In the United States, 79.1% of clinically active general surgeons practice in urban areas with a ratio of general surgeons per 100,000 persons at 6.53 compared with 4.67 per 100,000 in small rural areas of the nation and 4.23 per 100,000 in similar areas in rural Iowa.[3] This disparity may seem insignificant given there is no single accepted criterion of an adequate general surgeon to population ratio. Knowing that often the general surgeon practicing in rural areas serves as resident gastroenterologist, gyne-cologist, trauma surgeon, orthopedist, urologist, and critical care specialist, however, the disparity becomes much more significant. This phenomenon equates to a greater disparity of procedures per surgeon when comparing surgeons practicing in urban areas with rural areas.[4,8] It is unknown why most surgeons choose to practice in urban areas but one can assume that many factors come into play as this decision is made. Obvious differences in urban and rural communities, differences in reimbursement, isolation, spouse and family interests, and differences in work load and call responsi-bility are only a few of the many factors. Many of these factors are "fixed" in a rural surgery setting. Making a change in practice type can resolve some of the issues that are not necessarily "fixed," however, just because the surgical practice is within a rural community.

THE SOLUTION

Group practice is not usually something one thinks of when considering employment opportunities for general surgery in rural areas. Typically, surgeons practicing in rural areas do so independently. They describe their practices as isolated with little accountability from other surgeons. Call responsibility is usually significant and is a great challenge to spouse and family. Recruiting general surgeons to practice in rural areas has become increasingly difficult. Many young surgeons desire a lifestyle that is "more controllable" than that of a rural surgical practice.[9] The use of conventional group practice design, however, applied to IRSA has resolved many of these issues.

EVOLUTION OF A RURAL SURGICAL GROUP PRACTICE

IRSA was established in January of 2002 as a professional corporation with two board-certified general surgeons. The initial plan was to develop a surgical practice available to provide a broad range of surgical coverage to the community in and around Oskaloosa, Iowa, a community of approximately 10,000 people. In November of 2002, Ottumwa, a community approximately 30 miles southeast of Oskaloosa, lost their surgical coverage. IRSA was asked to provide coverage until that hospital was able to re-establish general surgery services in their community. Eight months later, IRSA was relieved of that commitment when that community successfully recruited a new general surgeon.

After helping the Ottumwa hospital, IRSA made a decision to be willing to provide temporary coverage for other surrounding communities if and when surgical coverage was lost. IRSA agreed to be reimbursed only for services rendered, to avoid additional financial burden for these communities in the midst of losing their surgical coverage, allowing IRSA freedom to provide assistance without being contractually bound to more than one institution.

Within 1 year, Pella, a nearby community of nearly 10,000 people, lost their surgical coverage. IRSA was once again asked to provide assistance. Because of the close proximity of Pella to Oskaloosa at only 16 miles, IRSA decided to hire an additional surgeon and start an IRSA satellite clinic in Pella. The solution to many logistical issues came in the form of the electronic medical record (EMR). With an EMR, billing could be centralized, charts could be made available at remote locations immediately, and IRSA could function as one in two separate communities. With the addition of a third surgeon in 2004, IRSA began to provide full-time surgical coverage in Oskaloosa and Pella. With the first two surgeons living in Oskaloosa, the third surgeon was located in Pella so that each community could reap the benefits of having a surgeon living and practicing in their own community.

Within 2 more years, Knoxville, a community of over 9000 people located 14 miles from Pella and 26 miles from Oskaloosa, lost their access to full-time general surgery coverage. IRSA once again decided to assist and recruited an additional surgeon to live and practice in the Knoxville community. The EMR allowed the fourth surgeon and the new clinic in the Knoxville Area Community Hospital to be "connected" with other IRSA clinics in Pella Regional Health Center in Pella and Mahaska Health Partnership in Oskaloosa.

To minimize full-time employees (FTE's), billing was centralized and office and nursing staff were trained to perform a wide variety of tasks. All clinics were designed to function similarly to facilitate shuffling of office and nursing staff as necessary to meet needs among all sites. In July of 2007, a fifth surgeon joined IRSA. This surgeon joined the practice in Pella to meet the increasing surgical demands in that community. With the addition of this surgeon, the general surgery needs of the areas in and around Knoxville, Oskaloosa, and Pella, Iowa, were met.

The three communities of Knoxville, Oskaloosa, and Pella are triangulated at 14-, 16-, and 26-mile driving distances. Population among the three locations is just under 30,000, total. The drawing area population is approximately 60,000 to 80,000 people. This includes people from other communities in surrounding counties and smaller communities in Marion County, where Knoxville and Pella are located, and in Mahaska County, where Oskaloosa is located.

THE HOSPITALS

All three hospitals are critical access hospitals. One of the hospitals functions as a county hospital and the other hospitals are private. There are one level 3 and two level 4 trauma centers among the group of hospitals. Two of the hospitals use community ambulance services and one hospital owns and operates its own service.

In all three hospitals combined, six operating rooms and five endoscopy suites are currently available. IRSA general surgeons typically have access to these rooms every day of the week, which enhances productivity. Anesthesia is provided by experienced certified registered nurse anesthetists at all hospitals. Operating room personnel are typically trained in all, which helps provide a wide variety of services, around the clock, with limited staff.

Most referring physicians work out of hospital-based clinics. Most clinics are provider-based but some exist as independent practices. Each emergency department (ED) is staffed with physicians 24 hours a day and one facility staffs a daytime urgent care clinic out of the ED. All hospitals house visiting physician clinics staffed by specialists providing services that each community's needs dictate. These physicians represent the specialties of cardiology, ear-nose-throat, oncology, vascular surgery, nephrology, urology, allergy and immunology, pulmonology, and pediatrics, among others.

Each hospital houses a full component of radiology and laboratory services. Multi-slice CT, MRI, ultrasound, fluoroscopy, and limited interventional radiology are also available at all locations. One hospital uses a full-time radiologist and the other two share radiology services with nearby communities. Two of the three hospitals have nuclear medicine departments and stereotactic biopsies are provided at each hospital. All departments use digital processing allowing films to be viewed remotely.

Pathology services are provided by a contracted group of pathologists from Des Moines, Iowa, who oversee laboratory services at each hospital. Specimens are sent by courier from the hospitals to the pathology laboratory daily. Results are typically available within 48 hours of collection. Pathologists are also available for frozen sections, when scheduled in advance.

Maintaining viable surgical services at each of the hospitals is essential for future growth at these institutions. Being able to provide surgeons to these communities in a sustainable way gives the governing bodies at each institution the confidence to grow their respective organizations. One of the hospitals that IRSA serves is now completing a large addition and renovation project. One of the other two facilities is preparing to break ground in the fall of 2009 on a similar project and the last facility is in the planning stages of a surgery department renovation.

THE SURGEONS

Of the five surgeons of IRSA, three are MDs and two are DOs. The average age is just over 42 years, which is younger than the state average of nearly 48 years.[6] Four surgeons are male and one is female. With percent female at 20%, the group exceeds the national average of females practicing in small or large rural areas at 6.1% and 7.3%, respectively.[3] Four of the surgeons started their surgical careers in rural communities and one joined IRSA after practicing in an urban surgical practice for 1 year.

One surgeon has been in practice in the area for 25 years and the remaining surgeons have been in practice for 22 years, combined. Three surgeons lived near the communities in the past, which influenced their decision to locate to the area. All surgeons are involved in community activities outside the practice of surgery and all are raising, or have raised, their families in this area.

All surgeons are board certified and can work independently in the operating room. Each surgeon welcomes the assistance of partners when desired and each appreciates the opportunity to assist when asked. Although all surgeons desire autonomy in decision making, accountability among surgeons remains, particularly when caring for each other's patients when on call.

PROCEDURES

All surgeons perform a wide variety of general surgery procedures in addition to cesarean sections; endoscopy; trauma; and a mixture of minor orthopedic, urologic, gynecologic, plastic surgery, and ear-nose-throat procedures. Training for this wide mix of procedures occurred intentionally, either during residency training or from mentoring within IRSA. None of the institutions have the resources for major vascular surgery and limited thoracic surgery is performed for the same reason. The exception includes emergency surgery or procedures in which transfer to tertiary care centers is not possible because of severe weather.

Average case numbers per surgeon is just under 900 per year. Endoscopy makes up approximately 50% of procedures followed by laparoscopy at 13%. Abdominal surgery and alimentary tract surgery follow at 7% each, with obstetrics next (mostly cesarean sections) at just under 6% of all cases. Gynecology, breast, and musculo-skeletal surgery follow at nearly 4% each, and genitourinary and orthopedic cases round out the remaining procedures at less than 3% each.

CLINICS

Each community has an IRSA clinic situated within the hospital located close to operating rooms and referring physician clinics. Clinic space is leased from each hospital. Contracts vary in length from 1 to 5 years and lease costs vary from $13.50 to nearly $30 per square foot, annually. Contracts vary significantly among hospitals, for a variety of reasons, despite overall similarities among facilities. IRSA assimilates differences that do exist among hospitals and strives to develop productive relationships with each institution. These relationships may not be exactly the same at each location, but maintaining healthy relationships with each facility allows IRSA the greatest opportunity to best serve the patients in these communities.

Ten nonsurgeon FTEs make up the IRSA staff. Five of these FTE's fulfill nursing duties pairing each surgeon with one nurse. The remaining employees take care of clerical, reception, and billing duties. One employee functions as clinic manager for all sites and another is the billing manager for all sites. The EMR facilitates information sharing between offices and streamlines the billing process. Days in accounts receivable have decreased from over 60 days to less than 45 days while growing the practice and maintaining a ratio of two FTEs per surgeon.

Office staff and physicians maintain intentional communication to allow daily processes to run as smooth as possible. Offices typically meet monthly by site, and all sites meet quarterly to review processes, establish action plans, and build unity among employees that work daily toward the same goals, albeit by remote locations. Surgeons meet monthly to review cases, arrange call schedules, and develop ongoing practice plans. Finally, surgeons meet quarterly with the business and billing manager to review financial records, set and adjust budgets, and address other necessary business issues.

CALL SCHEDULES

Call schedules for surgeons are arranged in 3-month blocks. There is always one surgeon on primary call for all communities nights and weekends. A second surgeon is always available as back-up and usually called only for emergent cases, such as cesarean sections, when the on-call surgeon is in surgery and unavailable. Call averages one in five weekends and one night per week. Weekend call runs Friday 6 PM until Monday 7 AM and weekday call from 6 PM until 7 AM the following morning. Weekday call is managed by surgeons at their respective hospitals. During every 3-month block of call (quarter), each surgeon keeps the same weeknight of call. This night changes every quarter and after five quarters, one surgeon goes off the rotation taking no weeknight call for a quarter. Back-up call is always the night before the primary on-call night. Holiday call is set in 5-year blocks, rotated, and includes back-up call. Any call schedule changes are the responsibility of the surgeon needing to make a change (ie, alerting hospitals, finding coverage, and so forth).

On-call responsibilities include ED consults, in-patient consults, trauma consults, and cesarean section coverage, at all three locations. The primary call surgeon follows postoperative patients at each hospital during the on-call period and "hands-off" patients to surgeons at their respective hospitals on the following weekday morning. A courtesy call or text message from the primary call surgeon to the receiving surgeon occurs shortly after the call period ends to alert of any on-call surgical activity.

Each surgical patient is followed and care managed primarily by IRSA surgeons. Assistance provided by family practitioners or internal medicine physicians occurs on a case-by-case basis, as needed. In the event of a need for reoperation, the primary surgeon is given first opportunity. If the patient was cared for by the on-call surgeon and "handed-off" to a partner surgeon, however, the partner surgeon who has been following the patient understands the primary surgeon may not be available at the time reoperation is needed, and assumes this responsibility, as necessary. Each surgeon typically rounds on their own patients at their respective hospital 7 days per week. The primary on-call surgeon is also available to see partner's patients as needed to cover for vacation or educational leave.

REFERRALS TO IRSA

IRSA sees referrals from a variety of sources. The most common sources include any of the approximately 25 family physicians that practice in the three communities plus referrals from several other family physicians in other surrounding communities. Referrals from EDs are also a significant source of referrals. Other sources include internal medicine physicians (approximately five); referrals from a variety of allied health professionals; and word-of-mouth referrals from prior patients (which typically come in the form of self-referrals). A significant number of referrals come from encounters with potential patients at church, sporting events, the county fair, hardware store, and the grocery store. Spouses, friends, and relatives of IRSA surgeons also keep a steady stream of patients coming to the clinics. Finally, the hospitals show their support of referrals to IRSA surgeons with frequent newspaper advertisements and public service announcements.

IRSA surgeons rarely refer patients to tertiary care hospitals. Typically, critically ill patients that need specialized care, or require resources not readily available in the local medical communities, are transferred. Examples include transfer of patients needing angiography, extended ventilator support, or inpatient dialysis. Trauma patients with severe neurologic or orthopedic injuries are always transferred and burn-injured patients are typically stabilized and transferred.

RECENT DEVELOPMENTS

Recently, IRSA considered the role of the group in the future. With five surgeons, coverage and call advantages are maximized. Tighter operating margins resulting from declining reimbursement and increased numbers of uninsured patients coupled with a continued desire by the surgeons to support the local medical communities, as surgeon partners, however, prompted a re-evaluation of the group plan. A decision was made to sell the practice of IRSA to each of the hospitals. When the hospitals were presented with this plan, each was eager to move ahead with the addition of a provider-based surgical practice at each location. All hospitals and surgeons wanted to take advantage of enhanced reimbursement benefits available to critical access hospitals when using their own physicians. As a result, all surgeons became employees of the hospitals in their own communities.

The only discernable difference has been receiving paychecks from the hospitals. The sale included selling all assets to each respective hospital. The EMR was sold to one of the hospitals and it remains in use at this location. The other two hospitals have implemented their own hospital-wide EMRs into IRSA offices. Billing personnel have been incorporated into hospital billing departments and nurses and clerical staff have been retained in the individual clinics.

Surgeons continue with the same call schedule and meetings are now only for the discussion of cases and planning call schedules. Referral patterns remain the same. IRSA surgeons and hospital administrations have addressed this change with the local medical communities to show surgical care in this region remains the same despite the sale of the private corporation. It is hoped that surgical care continues to improve in this region as this collaboration provides a new framework for the former surgeons of IRSA to continue their partnering work.

DISCUSSION

Rural surgeons have many choices within which to deliver surgical care in their respective communities. They can work alone or partner with other surgeons, as distance allows. They can be self-employed or hospital-employed. Work can be done at one or multiple hospitals. The possibilities are limited only by the imagination of the surgeon.

Rural communities benefit most from surgeons who perform a wide variety of procedures, are readily available, and are willing to work to maintain a sustainable practice. This means surgeons practicing in rural areas need to be flexible, well trained, and more motivated to serve than be served. This is a tall order particularly, when considering quality of life issues. Many surgeons no longer desire to make this commitment alone, and for this reason overlook rural general surgery practice opportunities. The group practice model often used in urban surgical practices can be applied to some rural areas in a way that can benefit both patients and surgeons. The only requirement is a willingness to partner with surgeons and hospitals of other communities.

Barriers exist that may make partnering in rural areas difficult. Many communities are simply too distant to facilitate this type of arrangement. For rural areas where distance is not limiting, community hospitals might compete with each other for the same patient population. Neighboring surgeons, unfortunately, can assume this same competitive relationship while simultaneously wishing they had surgical partners to share call and work responsibilities with, just like their "lucky" urban counterparts.

IRSA surgeons have learned partnering together can overcome the obstacles of competition among neighboring communities. The greatest benefit is improved care for surgical patients. Another is improved quality of life for rural surgeons who cooperate. Although quality of life is not the driving force for such a commitment, IRSA surgeons believe that surgical care of patients is better when the quality of life for surgeons in rural areas is improved. IRSA has shown how this can be accomplished as a group practice in the past. Furthermore, IRSA surgeons desire to realize this benefit now and in the future, as they continue to partner together to provide surgical care for patients in this region, despite the recent sale of the professional corporation.

SUMMARY

To say IRSA was developed as a model to improve the quality of life for rural surgeons is an overstatement. Improving surgical coverage in this area of southeast Iowa was the primary goal. The desire of the surgeons to extend themselves combined with the cooperation of their hospitals has resulted in improved surgical care for patients in this region. A by-product of this collaborative effort, however, has been improved quality of life for the surgeons and families of IRSA. To this end, things that have been done at IRSA can be replicated in other rural areas when surgeons and hospitals desire to work together to improve surgical coverage in their own communities. It is hoped that surgeon's quality of life also can be improved elsewhere.

REFERENCES

1. Kwakwa F, Jonasson O. The general surgery workforce. Am J Surg 1997;173: 59–62.
2. Landercasper J, Bintz M, Cogbill TH, et al. Spectrum of general surgery in rural America. Arch Surg 1997;132:494–6.
3. Thompson MJ, Lynge DC, Larson EH, et al. Characterizing the general surgery work-force in rural America. Arch Surg 2005;140:74–9.
4. Merchant JA, Rohrer JE, Urdaneta M, et al. Provision of comprehensive health care to rural Iowans in the 21st century. The University of Iowa Health of the Public Program, the University of Iowa; 1994.
5. Johna S. The rural surgeon: an endangered species. World J Surg 2006;30:267–8.
6. Shively E, Shively S. Threats to rural surgery. Am J Surg 2005;190:200–5.
7. Breon TA, Scott-Conner CEH, Tracy RD. Spectrum of general surgery in Iowa. Curr Surg 2003;60:94–9.
8. Ritchie WP, Rhodes RS, Biester TW. Work loads and practice patterns of general surgeons in the United States, 1995–1997, a report from the American Board of Surgery. Ann Surg 1999;230:533–43.
9. Bland KI, Isaacs G. Contemporary trends in student selection of medical special-ties. Arch Surg 2002;137:259–67.

Rural Surgery: The North Dakota Experience

David. R. Antonenko, MD, PhD, FRCS(C), FACS

KEYWORDS

- Rural surgery • Rural manpower • Surgical education
- Resident training • General surgery workforce

North Dakota is primarily a rural state with most of the counties classed as either rural or wilderness. There are 640,000 people residing in an area of 68,976 square miles for a population density of 9.3 people per square mile. Only three cities have a metropolitan population of over 50,000. The majority of the state's population lives in small or isolated rural areas. Native Americans are the largest minority in the state and account for 5.3% of the population. Almost 15% of state residents are elderly with a higher percentage of elderly in the rural areas. The state's elderly population, as in many regions of the country, is expected to grow for the foreseeable future. Since the need for surgery increases with age,[1] this increase in the elderly population will require a substantial increase in surgeons in the rural areas of the state. Many patients in small or isolated rural areas must commute distances of over 1 hour to see a surgeon. This commute may be much longer, or even impossible at times, because of inclement weather.

North Dakota is the only state in a four-state area that has a surgical residency. Montana, Wyoming, and South Dakota must obtain their surgeons from residency programs in other parts of the country. These states surrounding North Dakota to the south and west have demographics similar to North Dakota. With the exception of the large population centers in each of these states where surgery supply is adequate, smaller communities have few or no surgeons. In a recent survey of surgeons in the Dakotas, 57% of surgeons are over 50 years of age.[2] This will increase since recruiting surgeons to rural practice has become more difficult. Some smaller communities have been trying to recruit a surgeon for up to 5 years. Almost 60% of the smaller hospitals in North Dakota have stopped providing obstetrics coverage because of the loss of the general surgeon or the inability to recruit a surgeon. This exposes pregnant women and fetuses to increased risk at the time of delivery.

Nationally, there are a diminishing number of graduating residents who opt for careers in general surgery. Even fewer look to practice in rural sites. Recent data

Department of Surgery, University of North Dakota, School of Medicine & Health Sciences, Room 5108, 501 N. Columbia Road STOP 9037, Grand Forks, ND 58202-9037, USA
E-mail address: danton@medicine.nodak.edu

Surg Clin N Am 89 (2009) 1367–1372
doi:10.1016/j.suc.2009.07.010
0039-6109/09/$ – see front matter © 2009 Elsevier Inc. All rights reserved.

indicates almost 80% of current surgical residents elect fellowship training after general surgical residency.[3] Rural areas must compete for these graduates and, in many ways, are at a disadvantage because of location, reduced reimbursement, lack of peer support, a sense of isolation, and no or limited call coverage.[4] Urban training programs in general reflect the urban definition of general surgery (usually a restricted practice). Few residency programs provide training in general surgery that is specific for rural practice requirements. Although a few large residency programs have started a rural track for residents,[5] many surgeons practicing in rural areas have probably come from smaller community or community-based university programs such as the University of North Dakota (UND), Marshfield Clinic in Wisconsin, and Cooperstown in New York. These programs train residents for practice in smaller communities or rural areas.

Because of the rural nature of the state (and surrounding states) and the needs of rural or small communities, the surgical residency in North Dakota has always provided training for its residents that allows them to practice in smaller communities or rural areas. There is now general agreement that a shortage of general surgeons exists in the country, particularly in rural areas.[6] As of 2005, there were 7.7 surgeons per 100,000 people in the three urban areas of North Dakota, in contrast to a national average of 6.5 per 100,000 in urban areas. In large rural areas, North Dakota had 11.8 surgeons per 100,000 versus 7.7 per 100,000 nationally. In small rural areas, there were only 3.76 surgeons per 100,000 compared to 4.6 per 100,000 nationally. Many surgical patients from small or isolated rural areas are referred to large rural or urban areas for surgical care. This is a reflection of smaller hospitals in the state converting to critical access hospitals and increasing regionalization of surgical care because of the inability to recruit surgeons.

PROGRAM DEVELOPMENT

The UND School of Medicine and Health Sciences has been in existence for over 100 years. However, it was not until 1982 that a general surgery residency was started by Dr Edwin C. James, Chairman of the Department of Surgery. Under his leadership and with the support of the general surgeons in Grand Forks and other parts of the state, the first residents were recruited in 1982 and graduated in 1986. As of June 30, 2008, the residency program has graduated 44 residents and 18 (41%) continue to practice in rural or small communities. Initially the program graduated two residents per year but expanded to a three resident per year program in 2008. There are no other surgical trainees in the state of North Dakota, including obstetrics and gynecology or any of the surgical specialties. There are also no surgical fellowships in the Departments of Surgery or any hospital in North Dakota. This allows surgical residents almost unlimited access to all of general surgery cases and cases within surgical specialties. The initial surgical experiences for residents were developed according to Accreditation Council for Graduate Medical Education (ACGME) requirements in existence at the time the program started in 1982. These included dedicated rotations on anesthesiology; pathology; plastic and reconstructive surgery; orthopedics, ear, nose, and throat (ENT); and urology. These rotations were 2 or 3 months in length and were in Grand Forks and Fargo hospitals. Rotations in orthopedics, ENT, and urology (most at the Veterans Administration Hospital in Fargo) were particularly valuable for residents who were to practice in rural hospitals.

Pediatric surgery rotations were initially in Fargo but with the loss of this experience in 1995, an agreement with the Arnold Palmer Hospital for Women and Children in Orlando, Florida, provided our fourth-year residents a 2-month rotation on the pediatric surgery service. Having a more senior resident rotate on the service resulted in an excellent operative experience with many residents leaving the pediatric service having performed more than 100 minor and major pediatric operative cases.

Although the UND residents had experience in blunt trauma within the core teaching hospitals in North Dakota, experience in penetrating trauma was obtained through an affiliation agreement with University of California at San Francisco Fresno. The fourth-year residents from UND spent 3 months on the trauma service at this hospital from 1984 to 1996. In order to reduce travel time for residents and their families, in 2000 the trauma rotation was transferred to Orlando Regional Medical Center where the residents now rotate for 2 months on pediatric surgery and 2 months on the trauma service.

In keeping with the residency objectives, which incorporate experience in rural surgery, a 1-month experience in each of the first 2 years of residency was developed at the Belcourt Indian Health Services hospital on the Turtle Mountain Indian reservation in north central North Dakota. Residents not only evaluated patients and operated on them in Belcourt but also spent time in outpatient clinics on other reservations in North and South Dakota. These native Americans are one of the most impoverished ethnic minorities in the country. Under the supervision of a board certified general surgeon, residents performed a large number of basic surgical cases without competition from other residents. This rotation was funded by a grant from the Indian Health Service. Although the rotation was felt to have significant educational value for the junior residents, by 1995 grant funds were not sufficient to support the program and the rotation was stopped. Although residents continued to obtain training that would allow them to practice in small communities or in rural areas, a specific rural experience was not reinstated until 2003 when residents began rotating for 1 month with a board certified surgeon in a hospital in Park Rapids, Minnesota, which is a town with a population just over 3,000. This hospital is now a designated center of excellence for bariatric surgery. Many residents have performed over 100 surgical cases during their 1 month rotation, including many advanced laparoscopic cases.

All residents from the inception of the program have rotated through the Veterans Administration Medical Center in Fargo. This rotation provides them the opportunity to organize and run a service.

In addition, it provides them operative experience in simple and complex general surgery, urology, thoracic surgery, and, particularly, endoscopy. The latter training is very important for graduates who practice in rural or small communities because a substantial part of the practice of a rural surgeon is endoscopy.[7–9] The majority of graduates meet the requirements for basic endoscopy privileges as set by most national organizations including the Society of American Gastrointestinal and Endoscopic Surgeons.[10] The residents average over 250 endoscopies (range 100–300), with experience in both upper and lower endoscopy by the time they graduate.

Although not possible in large institutions where service to the general surgery rotation is a frequent requirement and competition with other residents and fellows in various surgery specialties is the norm, the UND program allows exposure to surgical specialties by incorporating them into the general surgical services. For example, ENT and urology are considered part of one service at Altru Hospital in Grand Forks and plastic surgery and thoracic surgery are considered part of another service. Residents are able to choose operative experiences in a number of surgical specialties on any given day.

Nephrectomies, ileal loops, thoracotomies, and other procedures such as rotation flaps, and head and neck procedures historically considered part of general surgery are cases performed by the senior residents without interfering with their experience in general surgery. Should a resident request a specific experience in other specialties that may be required in their chosen practice location, this is arranged during the general surgery rotations in their fourth and fifth years. Several residents have had additional exposure to Caesarian sections, as they would be expected to perform them in the practices they entered after graduation. The author thinks that a surgical experience that will allow exposure to areas specific to a practice requirement, particularly rural or small community practice, is attainable within current Residency Review Committee (RRC) guidelines if the program is structured properly.

The Department of Surgery has had no more than four full-time surgical faculty at any time. Almost all teaching of medical students and residents is done by part-time or volunteer clinical faculty that is similar to the preceptorship, mentor program recently reported for Swedish Medical Center in Seattle, Washington.[11] Of the 1300 cases performed on average by our residents, over 90% are completed by the resident as primary surgeon under the supervision of the volunteer faculty. Exposure to clinical faculty with diverse backgrounds in training provides residents with varied experiences in academic, community, and rural practices. Most of our residents have listed over 300 operative procedures as primary surgeon by the end of their second year, as many as junior residents in many urban programs where operative experience in the first 2 years of residency is limited.

MEDICAL STUDENTS AND THE SURGICAL RESIDENCY

The surgical residency program has been involved in undergraduate medical student education since the start of the program. Resident involvement includes proctoring in the anatomy cadaver lab where they teach anatomy to first-year medical students, and facilitating case discussions in the second-year patient centered learning (PCL) blocks. A surgical interest group was developed to provide students in the first 2 years of medical school exposure to multiple surgical specialties, including general surgery. These students also participate in clinical teaching rounds. Third-year students are provided exposure to urology, ENT, and cardiovascular surgery. In the fourth year, they have a mandatory 2 week orthopedic surgery rotation as part of their 4th year one month acting internship.

Table 1
Residency selection as percent of class year, (class size), and total graduates selecting each specialty (others include radiology, dermatology, etc)

Specialty	2002 (53)	2003 (53)	2004 (54)	2005 (50)	2006 (54)	2007 (54)	2008 (62)	2009 (61)
Family medicine	22.6	7.5	18.5	20.0	11.0	7.2	27.4	15.3
Internal medicine	11.3	9.4	13.0	12.0	13.2	13.2	9.8	13.6
Obstetrics and gynecology	13.2	11.3	9.3	14.0	9.4	9.4	6.6	11.9
Pediatrics	9.4	7.5	5.6	10.0	17.0	17.0	9.8	11.9
General surgery	11.3	18.9	5.6	6.0	15.1	15.1	11.5	15.3
All surgical specialties	18.9	30.3	15.1	18.0	22.7	22.7	21.3	20.7
Emergency medicine	7.5	7.5	13.0	12.0	5.7	5.7	13.1	6.8
Other	5.8	7.6	22.2	8.0	21.9	20.7	0.7	4.5

Table 2 University of North Dakota, general surgery residency graduates[a]			
	Total	Rural	Urban
General surgery	29	17	12
Plastic surgery	3	1	2
Cardio thoracic	3	0	3
Vascular	3	1	2

[a] One fellowship in each of pediatric surgery, colorectal, trauma, surgical oncology, minimally invasive, and transplant surgery.

Third and fourth year medical students are dispersed throughout the state for their clinical rotations but must participate in residency morbidity and mortality conferences and surgery grand rounds, with the use of video-conferencing. The one-on-one preceptorship with faculty has been the basis, not only for a high percentage of the class entering a surgical specialty (**Table 1**), but also for a high proportion of those pursuing rural or community practice when they graduate. This is in keeping with previous literature on the subject.[12] Of the 15 UND School of Medicine graduates who have finished the UND general surgical residency, seven (47%) continue to practice in rural areas.

Table 2 reflects the practice choice of graduates of the general surgery residency. In contrast to the national trend of graduates increasingly pursuing fellowship training, only 15 of the 44 graduates (36%) from our residency have pursued fellowships and two of them practice in rural areas of various states. Of the 29 general surgeons who did not take fellowship training, 17, or 58% practice in rural sites.

SUMMARY

In a study looking at surgeons in health service areas, Finlayson[13] reported that 20% of urban areas and 21% of large rural areas reported a low supply of surgeons. However, 39% of small rural health supply areas and 66% of isolated rural areas reported problems with surgeon availability. There is, and has been for some years, a crisis regarding rural surgery that is unrecognized or ignored by major teaching programs and major surgical organizations with the exception perhaps of the American College of Surgeons. Unless there is a drastic increase in the supply of surgeons who are appropriately trained for rural areas, patients' lack of access will result in delays in care and increased transport distances, which may jeopardize patient care particularly in emergency situations. The American Board of Surgery, the ACGME, and surgery RRCs must allow programs to change dramatically from the time-honored, locked-in rotations that have been prevalent in urban training programs for decades. The Blue Ribbon Committee report from the American Surgical Association[14] is frequently quoted with respect to the direction general surgery resident training should take; but the dissenting opinion by two pillars of the surgical community that support distinct training for urban and rural general surgeons must be recognized.[15] General surgery programs should be encouraged and allowed to be innovative and not penalized for adjusting their programs to allow residents to train for rural and community sites.

Although the basics of surgery should still be the foundation of general surgery training, latitude must be provided to programs so they can provide training for surgical residents that will meet the needs of all people and not just the urban areas of the country. There must be increased support for training, continuing education, and support for surgeons in rural communities and less criticism of care if outcomes of surgical specialty care are not 100% equal to these elite surgical groups.

Surgeons in rural and community sites need to document their experiences and compare them with larger institutions.

Participation in the American College of Surgeons National Surgical Quality Improvement Program and case log programs is strongly encouraged. Experiences of individual practices must be examined for quality and safety. Quality of care must be acceptable in all sites but the attitudes and perceptions of large training programs and specialty organizations based only on urban studies should not be applied universally until fully researched.

The general surgery residency program at UND continues to provide the best training consistent with the practice requirements of its graduates—particularly those who chose to practice in smaller community and rural sites.

REFERENCES

1. Etzioni DA, Liu JH, Maggard MA, et al. The aging population and its impact on the surgery workforce. Ann Surg 2003;238(2):170–7.
2. Harris, J, Sticca, R. Rural surgery in the upper Midwest: a descriptive survey. Rural Surgery Symposium, Grand Forks, ND, submitted to Journal of the American College of Surgeons, September 2009.
3. Borman K, Vick LR, Biester TW, et al. Changing demographics of residents choosing fellowships: longterm data from the American board of surgery. J Am Coll Surg 2008;206:782–9.
4. Shively EH, Shively SA. Threats to rural surgery. Am J Surg 2005;190:200–5.
5. Hunter JG, Deveney KE. Training the rural surgeon: a proposal. Bull Am Coll Surg 2003;88(5):13–7.
6. Lynge DC, Larson EH, Thompson MJ, et al. A longitudinal analysis of the general surgery workforce in the United States, 1981–2005. Arch Surg 2008;143(4):345–50.
7. Landercasper J, Bintz M, Cogbill TH, et al. Spectrum of general surgery in rural America. Arch Surg 1997;132(5):494–7.
8. Heneghan SJ, Bordley J, Dietz PA, et al. Comparison of urban and rural general surgeons: motivations for practice location, practice patterns, and education requirements. J Am Coll Surg 2005;201(5):732–6.
9. Zuckerman R, Doty B, Bark K, et al. Rural versus non-rural differences in surgeon performed endoscopy: results of a national survey. Am Surg 2007;73(9):903–5.
10. Society of American Gastrointestinal and Endoscopic Surgeons. Granting of privileges for gastrointestinal endoscopy, September 2007. Available at: www.sages.org. Accessed April 22, 2009.
11. Hart M. Presidential address. Lessons learned from 25 years as a surgery residency program director. Am J Surg 2009;197:553–6.
12. Asher EF, Martin MD. Rural rotations for senior surgical residents. Arch Surg 1984;119:1120–4.
13. Finlayson S. Access to surgery in rural America, Rural Surgery Symposium, Grand Forks (ND). Available at: www.med.und.nodak.edu/surgery/documents/symposium/Finlayson-AccesstoSurgery.ppt. September 2007. Accessed May 14, 2009.
14. Debas HT, Bass BL, Brennan ME, et al. American Surgical Association Blue Ribbon Committee report on surgical education. Ann Surg 2005;241(1):1–8.
15. Brennan MF, Debas HT. Surgical education in the United States: portents for change. Ann Surg 2004;240:565–72.

Assessing and Improving the Quality of Surgical Care in Rural America

Samuel R.G. Finlayson, MD, MPH[a,b,c,*]

KEYWORDS

• Quality of care • Quality improvement • Rural surgery

Amidst the many ideas, opinions, and debates currently swirling in the public forum on health care policy, the most consistent theme is the call for improvement in the quality of care. The Institute of Medicine articulated this theme in the publication *Crossing the Quality Chasm*, calling for health care that is safer, more effective, more efficient, more equitable, more patient-centered, and more timely.[1] Efforts to improve the quality of health care represent the convergence of many interests: the patients' interest in achieving the best possible health, the health care providers' interest in their patients' outcomes and in building successful practices in a competitive market, and the payers' interest in avoiding the costs associated with poor health care.[2] It is no surprise, therefore, that reform and improvement of the quality of health care has become a top national priority.

Efforts to understand and improve the quality of surgical care are not new, but have gained greater urgency as the quality of health care has assumed greater prominence in the public consciousness. In addition to the longstanding tradition of local peer review of surgical morbidity and mortality, there is a fast-growing body of articles reporting the results of research in surgical outcomes. At an institutional level, several significant and high-profile surgical quality initiatives have emerged in the last two decades, including the American College of Surgeons National Surgical Quality Improvement Program (ACS-NSQIP, developed initially in the Veterans Administration and then extrapolated to the public sector),[3] the Leapfrog Group's surgical care initiatives, Surgical Care Improvement Program (SCIP),[4] the Michigan Plan,[5] and the Surgical Care Outcomes Assessment Program.[6]

[a] Department of Surgery, Dartmouth-Hitchcock Medical Center, 1 Medical Center Drive, Lebanon, NH 03756, USA
[b] The Dartmouth Institute for Health Policy and Clinical Practice, 35 Centerra Parkway, Lebanon, NH 03766, USA
[c] The Mithoefer Center for Rural Surgery, 1 Atwell Street, Cooperstown, NY 13326, USA
* Dartmouth-Hitchcock Medical Center, 1 Medical Center Drive, Lebanon, NH 03756.
E-mail address: srgf@hitchcock.org

Surg Clin N Am 89 (2009) 1373–1381
doi:10.1016/j.suc.2009.09.013   surgical.theclinics.com
0039-6109/09/$ – see front matter © 2009 Elsevier Inc. All rights reserved.

Although efforts to improve surgical quality are effectively addressing the conditions of larger urban and suburban hospitals, they are less easily applied to smaller hospitals, many of which are in rural areas of the United States. Already, there is public suspicion that small rural hospitals may not provide high-quality care. Small rural hospitals' problems of public perception are further compounded when new surgical quality standards and programs seem beyond their reach.

This article describes some of the challenges related to applying surgical quality assessment and improvement initiatives to the practice of surgery in small rural hospitals. These challenges must be met because rural residents will continue to require the services of surgeons in rural hospitals, and the care that these surgeons provide must necessarily be of the highest possible quality. This article also presents approaches to addressing these challenges to stimulate dialog about surgical quality improvement in small rural hospitals.

BARRIERS TO QUALITY ASSESSMENT OF RURAL SURGERY

There are numerous barriers to the implementation of surgical quality assessment techniques and quality improvement measures in small rural hospitals. These include professional isolation, limited financial and other resources, low surgical volume, and differences between urban and rural populations.

Professional Isolation

Even before health care quality became a national priority and quality assessment and improvement achieved a higher level of sophistication, keeping a close watch to identify and prevent the repetition of surgical errors was a challenge in small rural hospitals. The traditional approach to surgical quality assessment and improvement is the surgical morbidity and mortality conference (M&M conference), a private meeting regularly convened by surgeons to review bad outcomes and identify what went wrong, what mistakes might have been made, and how similar outcomes might be avoided in the future. In a large urban hospital, this process involves many surgeons with extensive combined experience. In a small rural hospital, however, peer review is typically limited to very few surgeons (or even just one surgeon) and a few nonsurgeons. Thus even at the most basic level in rural hospitals, the effectiveness of quality assessment and improvement through peer review is hampered by a disadvantage of numbers.

Insofar as quality is also measured by the degree to which the latest and best technologies and techniques are applied in surgical practice, small rural hospitals function at a disadvantage. First, because some new technologies are very expensive, small rural hospitals are unable to invest the capital required to acquire them. For example, sentinel node biopsy for breast cancer requires special capabilities and equipment, and their purchase is difficult to justify given the small number of patients with breast cancer presenting annually at a small rural hospital. Secondly, because of limited surgical staffing in rural hospitals, it is difficult to arrange time away from work for continuing medical education, and this can result in slower dissemination of new techniques and practices. Although Kemp and colleagues[7] reported that these barriers did not affect the time taken to adopt laparoscopic cholecystectomy, these challenges that are related to maintaining the state of the art in surgery are a core concern expressed by rural surgeons in forums addressing rural surgery practice.[8]

Low Volume

The association between higher volume of procedures and better surgical outcomes has been demonstrated repeatedly in medical literature. Although this association has been questioned,[9,10] the preponderance of statistical evidence supports the volume-outcome effect for many surgical procedures. The question is not whether the volume-outcome effect is real, but rather whether it is reasonable to use volume as a measure of quality and whether it is fair to use it as a justification for selective referral (regionalization).[11]

A false interpretation of the volume-outcome effect is the assumption that what is observed in the aggregate also holds true for specific cases. In other words, it is incorrect to assume that because low-volume hospitals have higher overall mortality than high-volume hospitals, all low-volume hospitals produce worse outcomes. The only valid conclusion about individual hospitals that one can draw from the volume-outcome effect is that the odds of choosing a hospital with good outcomes are higher when one chooses a high-volume hospital. However, there are certainly poor-performing high-volume hospitals and high-performing low-volume hospitals.

Volume is an ineffective measure of quality in small rural hospitals because most rural hospitals perform low volumes of the surgical procedures for which the volume-outcome effect has been demonstrated. Because most rural hospitals perform relatively low volumes of surgical procedures, the whole range of surgical quality, from low to high, may be represented. This hypothesis is supported by an analysis of Medicare claims data that Meyers and the author made several years ago. The study compared mortality rates in rural versus urban hospitals in the United States for colectomy for cancer, a procedure for which there is a demonstrated, significant volume-outcome effect.[12] The subjects for the study were drawn from all non-HMO Medicare claims for patients older than 65 years during a 6-year period (1994–1999). Urban and rural hospital designations were based on rural-urban commuting area (RUCA) codes developed by health services researchers at the University of Washington.[13] Multiple logistic regression was used to describe the relationship between combined in-hospital and 30-day mortality and the rural/urban hospital location, controlling for patient and hospital characteristics.

In the complete cohort of hospitals, the authors observed the same significant volume-outcome effect that was reported in a previous Medicare-based study of colectomy mortality.[14] However, the overall adjusted operative mortality in rural hospitals (6.7%; 95% confidence interval [CI], 6.4–7.0) was similar to that of urban hospitals (6.4%; 95% CI, 6.3–6.5), even though nearly 90% of rural hospitals were in the lowest 2 quintiles of hospital procedure volume (<57 colectomies/year) compared with only 28% of urban hospitals. When comparing adjusted operative mortality in the lowest 2 quintiles of hospital volume, it was found that mortality in the low-volume rural hospitals (6.6%; 95% CI, 6.3–6.9%) was significantly lower than mortality in urban hospitals with similar annual volume of procedures (7.2%; 95% CI, 7.0–7.4%).

In summary, nearly 90% of rural hospitals where colectomy for cancer is performed are low-volume hospitals, but their adjusted operative mortality is significantly lower than that of urban hospitals with similar procedure volume. Rural hospitals, although predominantly low volume, had an overall mortality rate that more closely resembled the overall mortality rate observed in the entire cohort of urban hospitals (**Fig. 1**). This finding may be explained by the presence of more low-volume high performers in the cohort of rural hospitals.

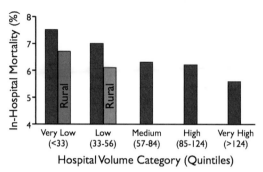

Fig. 1. Adjusted combined in-hospital and 30-day mortality after colectomy for cancer in Medicare (age>65 years) patients, 1994 to 1999. Black bars indicate urban hospital mortality across quintiles of hospital volume. Gray bars indicate mortality in low-volume rural hospitals (90% of all rural hospitals are in the 2 lowest quintiles).

As volume is an ineffective standard for quality in rural hospitals (because most are low-volume hospitals), the obvious alternative approach to identify the better performing hospitals is the direct measurement of surgical outcomes. However, the tendency for rural hospitals to perform relatively low volumes of surgical procedures presents an impediment to this approach. The reason for this is the low statistical power resulting from the small number of procedures in rural hospitals. When the number of outcomes (eg, mortality) being measured is low, statistical comparisons result in wide confidence intervals. This makes outcomes-based quality comparisons across hospitals very difficult for most procedures. This statistical problem exists not only for rural hospitals but also for most urban hospitals across various procedures, as demonstrated in an elegant analysis by Dimick and colleagues[15] published in 2004.

As a simple example, assume that during a given time period, procedures performed in a given region number 50,000, with 1500 deaths, yielding a benchmark mortality rate of 3%. Then assume that Hospital A during the same time period performed 46 procedures, with 4 deaths, yielding a mortality rate of 8%. Although this mortality rate would appear to be more than twice as high as the benchmark, conventional statistical comparison techniques (chi-square analysis) would suggest that the mortality rates are actually similar (no statistically significant difference). Now assume that Hospital B performed the same number of procedures as Hospital A, but with no deaths, yielding a mortality rate of 0%. Although Hospital B might consider these results exceptional, conventional statistical analysis again suggests no difference from the benchmark. As can be seen from this simple example, when bad outcomes are rare, outcomes-based quality assessment by conventional statistical methods is not adequate. Small rural hospitals with low surgical volumes are unable to distinguish themselves statistically as providing either superior or inferior quality of surgical care, based on analysis of outcomes.

Rural-Urban Patient Mix Differences

Largely on an anecdotal basis, it is believed that people who reside in rural areas are more prone to poor surgical outcomes because of comorbid medical conditions, more advanced disease, and socioeconomic factors. Although the protest "my patients are sicker" is a common complaint among providers faced with evidence of less-than-ideal surgical outcomes, it is certainly possible that regional population differences influence patient outcomes significantly. Although a small amount of research suggests that rural residents are not "sicker" on average,[16] the demand that outcomes analysis take into consideration patient differences is widely accepted, and risk adjustment is now considered standard practice in outcomes research and assessments of quality of care.

Risk adjustment for patient differences presents 2 important problems for rural surgery. The first relates to the intrinsic limitations of performing risk adjustment. Accounting for differences in populations requires the ability to accurately measure those differences. Accuracy of measurement in turn depends on the fidelity of the processes put in place to collect risk information, which may be subject to human error or information bias. Also, lists of comorbid conditions do not perfectly reflect true risk (eg, 2 patients with the same diabetes diagnosis may present very different risks). When comparing large populations, these limitations are less important, as the biases can work in either direction and tend to regress to a population mean. In rural practice, however, volumes are lower and thus more subject to the effects of random variation. When the cohort is small, a few patients who are at a high level of risk that is not well-reflected in the list of patient factors assigned to them can more easily skew results despite statistical risk adjustment. The second problem with risk adjustment when comparing smaller populations with fewer adverse outcomes relates to statistical confidence. Although risk adjustment is important for comparing populations that differ in baseline risk, it also widens statistical confidence intervals and results in diminished ability to discriminate between rates of adverse outcomes across comparison groups, particularly when the comparison groups are small and adverse outcomes are rare.

Fairness

What is most disconcerting for rural surgeons hampered by low procedure volumes is the sense that despite awareness of its limitations as a measure of quality in the rural setting, procedure volume continues to be a component of quality assessment and payer policy. Ease of measurement ensures the inclusion of procedure volume in hospital quality assessments issued to consumers by popular third party entities such as HealthGrades.[17] As another example, bariatric surgery is increasingly restricted to hospitals certified as centers of excellence, a category that requires a specific minimum in procedure volume.[18] Even if superior quality of care were demonstrable through direct outcomes measurement, most rural surgeons who want to include bariatric surgery in their practices would be prevented from doing so because of volume requirements. Whether high quality can truly be achieved in the setting of low volume may be an open question, but there is little doubt that many rural surgeons consider such policies unfair.

APPROACHES TO QUALITY ASSESSMENT AND IMPROVEMENT IN RURAL SETTINGS

Quality assessment and improvement in rural settings requires approaches that take into account the lower procedure volumes typical of a small rural hospital. Although problems with many current approaches persist, there have been several positive developments in the assessment and improvement of surgical quality. First, there is a growing recognition that in addition to outcomes, better processes in surgical care must be identified and implemented to improve surgical quality. Second, there are growing efforts to create and develop multi-institutional consortiums focused on improving the quality of surgical care. These efforts pay greater attention to the specific conditions of rural practice. Third, there is increasing recognition that a surgical workforce shortage in rural areas contributes to professional isolation and also bars access to surgical care, thereby diminishing the quality of care available to rural residents. Finally, efforts to understand the concept of "appropriate care" promise to improve quality in rural settings by helping surgeons understand who should receive what operations in what setting.

Focus on Processes of Care

One of the most consistent criticisms of early quality improvement programs was their overemphasis on outcomes. When the information gathered by a quality improvement program simply identifies hospitals with poor outcomes, there is no clear path to improvement. On the other hand, if processes of care (eg, appropriate use of antibiotics, use of appropriate technologies) are the metric by which quality is measured, the quality assessment itself clearly points to the changes required to improve quality.

In rural settings where low procedure volume stymies efforts to assess quality based on outcomes, quality is more appropriately assessed by determining the use of best practices. This approach obviates the problem of inadequate statistical power, as the benchmark for processes that should always be in place is 100% compliance. Outcomes in low volume settings cannot be interpreted with confidence, but they can be expected to reflect the benefits that a particular process of care has provided in clinical trials.

Process-based quality assessment and improvement has in recent years begun to gain momentum, notably with the development of SCIP and with proposed changes in the ACS-NSQIP.[19] SCIP is a widely accepted national quality improvement effort with a clear emphasis on a short list of easily measurable and effective processes of care, including prophylactic antibiotic use, appropriate hair removal technique, perioperative β-blocker use, maintenance of postoperative normothermia, and prophylaxis against deep venous thrombosis. The effort benefits from the partnership of private and public entities with a shared interest in improving the quality of surgical care. The ACS-NSQIP is a well-established and widely disseminated quality improvement program that has traditionally based quality assessment on risk-adjusted outcomes. Although this has been successful, there has been greater recognition in recent years of the need to add measurement of processes of care to this program, both as a means to assess hospital quality and a way to identify target areas for quality improvement.[19]

Although the assessment of processes of care has clear theoretical advantages, there are important practical limitations to this approach. Surgical care is complex and difficult to separate into individual independent processes. There is a lack of identifiable, scientifically based, universally accepted processes of care in surgery. Nevertheless, assessment of process of care remains the most promising quality assessment and improvement approach in low-volume rural settings. Unfortunately, there are few process-based quality improvement efforts such as SCIP, and they provide only a piecemeal approach to improving the quality of surgical care.

Quality Consortiums

Professional isolation in rural settings can be at least partially addressed by participation in consortiums focused on assessing and improving surgical quality. A successful example of this approach to quality improvement is the Surgical Care Outcomes Assessment Program (SCOAP).[6] SCOAP is a physician-led, voluntary, collaborative surgical quality program that aims to improve quality by reducing variations in processes of care in the Washington State region. Although participant hospitals are mostly larger urban and community hospitals, smaller hospitals meeting very minimal volume requirements are also encouraged to participate. The advantages of participation include the "surveillance and response" approach used by the consortium, which provides valuable opportunities for external peer review and has the potential to diminish the challenges related to professional isolation in rural practice.

Participation in the ACS-NSQIP can provide similar benefits, but at present, the cost and resource commitment required to enroll in the ACS-NSQIP has been a barrier for small rural hospitals with limited resources. Fortunately, the ACS-NSQIP is undertaking measures to streamline the program and make it more accessible to smaller institutions with limited resources. There is also discussion in the American College of Surgeons of creating a "lite" version of the ACS-NSQIP tailored for small rural hospitals (Clifford Ko, Director of the Division of Research and Optimal Patient Care, American College of Surgeons, personal communication).

Workforce

There is a heightened awareness of the shortage of general surgeons in rural areas.[20,21] The American College of Surgeons has played a key role in bringing invaluable political attention to the issue, and has made the rural workforce shortage a primary focus of its newly formed Health Policy Institute at the University of North Carolina. In response to these efforts (and the efforts of several other organizations concerned about physician workforce levels), the US Congress is presently considering legislation to address the barriers to increasing the workforce of physicians.

Although increasing the rural surgical workforce to provide rural residents with better access to surgical care is a laudable goal, simply increasing the overall number of trained general surgeons in the United States addresses this issue in the wrong way. The surgical workforce is unevenly distributed across the urban/rural spectrum, with lower overall surgeon-to-population ratios evident in most rural areas.[21] If the approach to rectifying shortages in rural areas is to significantly increase the national supply of surgeons, it is inevitable that the most attractive health care markets will have to be supersaturated before rural areas get relief. Insofar as oversupply is associated with increased health care costs with no corresponding incremental improvement in quality, the cost-effectiveness of surgical care can be expected to diminish in more populated oversupplied areas before the benefits of improved access are realized in less-populated rural areas. The public interest would be better served by specific policy measures to address the shortages in deficit areas. These measures might include targeted incentives, such as loan cancellation for residency graduates choosing to practice in under-served locales, or graduated reimbursement rates favoring rural practice. Such measures would significantly diminish the number of additional surgeons required to address the needs of areas short of surgeons in the United States.

Appropriateness of Surgical Care

Appropriateness, which is increasingly acknowledged as an important component of surgical quality, has special relevance to rural surgery. Although appropriateness is frequently used in reference to decisions about who should get what operation, in a broader sense appropriateness also refers to who should provide the operation, and in what setting.

For some higher risk procedures (eg, bariatric surgery), payers have taken the initiative by setting standards for reimbursement of hospitals, which effectively limit the hospitals where these operations are performed. In contrast, rural general surgeons are reluctant to set explicit limits on the scope of practice, and hospitals are often liberal in granting privileges, as limiting surgical practice has the potential to diminish revenue. However, the high degree of variability in outcomes for specific procedures across hospitals and surgeons suggests that some limits should exist. Even when an individual surgeon has the technical skill to perform a procedure well, the hospital setting can influence the eventual outcome substantially, as reported in a large study of pancreatic surgery that showed similar intraoperative morbidity rates in hospitals with very different rates of surgical mortality.[22] Although most would agree that there should be at least some limits on the scope of surgical procedures performed in rural hospitals with limited resources, it remains unclear where those limits should be fixed. Although we know that there are de facto differences between rural and urban hospital case mixes,[23] a more explicit evidence-based effort to define the appropriate scope of surgical practice in rural settings could add substantially to the quality of rural surgical care.

SUMMARY

The quality of surgical care in rural hospitals is important, as surgery remains a critical component of rural health care systems.[24] Current models for surgical quality assessment and improvement largely reflect the characteristics of larger urban hospital settings, which include proximity to other providers for peer review, higher procedure volumes to accurately assess outcomes, and greater financial resources to acquire data collection systems and finance participation in regional or national quality improvement programs such as the ACS-NSQIP. Although rural surgeons and hospitals face numerous challenges in their efforts to demonstrate or improve the quality of their surgical practices, developments in surgical quality favor their increased participation in quality improvement initiatives.

REFERENCES

1. Committee of Quality of Health Care in America, Institute of Medicine. Crossing the quality chasm: a new system for the 21st century. Washington, DC: The National Academies Press; 2001.
2. Dimick JB, Weeks WB, Karia RJ, et al. Who pays for poor surgical quality? Building a business case for quality improvement. J Am Coll Surg 2006;202: 933–7.
3. Fink AS, Campbell DA, Mentzer RM, et al. The national surgical quality improvement program in non-veterans administration hospitals: initial demonstration of feasibility. Ann Surg 2002;236:344–53.
4. SCIP Project Information. Available at: http://www.qualitynet.org/dcs/ContentServer?c=MQParents&pagename=Medqic/Content/ParentShellTemplate&cid=1122904930422&parentName=Topic. Accessed September 9, 2009.
5. Birkmeyer NJ, Share D, Campbell DA, et al. Partnering with payers to improve surgical quality: the Michigan Plan. Surgery 2005;138(5):815–20.
6. Flum DR, Fisher N, Thompson J, et al. Washington State's approach to variability in surgical processes/outcomes: Surgical Clinical Outcomes Assessment Program (SCOAP). Surgery 2005;138(5):821–8.
7. Kemp J, Zuckerman RA, Finlayson SRG. Trends in adoption of laparoscopic cholecystectomy in rural vs. urban hospitals. J Am Coll Surg 2008;206:28–32.
8. For the past 5 years, a forum for rural surgeons has been held at the Clinical Congress of the American College of Surgeons (ACS), sponsored by ACS Division of Member Services. A biannual Rural Surgery Symposium also provides an open forum for rural surgeons.

9. Khuri SF, Daley J, Henderson W, et al. Relation of surgical volume to outcome in eight common operations: results from the VA National Surgical Quality Improvement Program. Ann Surg 1999;230:414.
10. Wade TP, Halaby IA, Stapleton DR, et al. Population-based analysis of treatment of pancreatic cancer and Whipple resection: Department of Defense hospitals, 1989–1994. Surgery 1996;120:680–5.
11. Finlayson SRG. The volume-outcome debate revisited. Am Surg 2006;72: 1038–42.
12. Meyers, MA, SRG Finlayson. Should rural residents with colon cancer travel to urban hospitals for colectomy? Abstract presented at the Surgical Forum at the Clinical Congress of the American College of Surgeons. San Francisco, October 18, 2005.
13. WWAMI Rural Health Research Center. Rural-urban commuting area codes. Available at: http://depts.washington.edu/uwruca/. Accessed September 28, 2009.
14. Birkmeyer JD, Siewers AE, Finlayson EVA, et al. Hospital volume and surgical mortality in the United States. N Engl J Med 2002;346:1128–37.
15. Dimick JB, Welch HG, Birkmeyer JD. Surgical mortality as an indicator of hospital quality: the problem with small sample size. JAMA 2004;292:847–51.
16. Paquette I, Finlayson SRG. Rural versus urban colorectal and lung cancer patients: differences in stage at presentation. J Am Coll Surg 2007;205:636–41.
17. Healthgrades. Available at: http://www.healthgrades.com/. Accessed September 9, 2009.
18. Surgical Review Corporation. Bariatric surgery center of excellence requirements. Available at: http://www.surgicalreview.org/pcoe/tertiary/tertiary_provisional.aspx. Accessed September 9, 2009.
19. Birkmeyer JD, Shahian DM, Dimick JB, et al. Blueprint for a new American College of Surgeons-National Surgical Quality Improvement Program. Surgery 2008;207:777–82.
20. Cofer JB, Burns RP. The developing crisis in the national general surgery workforce. J Am Coll Surg 2008;206:790–7.
21. Thompson MJ, Lynge D, Larsen E, et al. Characterizing the general surgery workforce in rural America. Arch Surg 2005;140:74–9.
22. Glasgow RE, Mulvihill SJ. Hospital volume influences outcome in patients undergoing pancreatic resection for cancer. West J Med 1996;165(5):294–300.
23. Van Bibber M, Zuckerman R, Finlayson SRG. Rural versus urban inpatient case-mix differences in the United States. J Am Coll Surg 2005;201(3S):S76.
24. Doty BC, Zuckerman R, Finlayson SRG, et al. General surgery at rural hospitals: a national survey of rural hospital administrators. Surgery 2008;143:599–606.

General Surgery Contributes to the Financial Health of Rural Hospitals and Communities

Brit Doty, MPH[a], Steven J. Heneghan, MD[b,*], Randall Zuckerman, MD[a,c]

KEYWORDS

• Surgery • Rural • Economic contribution

It is intuitively recognized that rural residents benefit from access to local surgical care, but that rural hospitals may also profit from providing surgical services is less commonly acknowledged. Confirming this impression, most rural hospital administrators surveyed for several research studies perceived the ability to provide surgical care as very important to the financial viability and stability of their institutions.[1–3] Little research has been conducted that examined or quantified the specific economic contribution that a general surgeon or surgical services make to rural hospitals and communities. This article outlines what is known on this topic and focuses on the economic impact that surgical care delivery can have on rural hospitals and communities and the potential costs associated with not having a general surgeon or surgical services available at rural hospitals. The authors also discuss the financial limitations that rural hospitals face in providing surgical care and the economic impact of variations in the delivery of surgical care in different types of rural communities. In addition, questions for future research in this area are identified.

Rural hospitals provide valuable health care services for their communities while facing unique challenges, including coping with limited financial and human resources, as they respond to varying patient needs and expectations. Although the ability to offer a broad range of services may strengthen a rural hospital's financial condition, it can

Funding for the Mithoefer Center and this article was received from the Robert Keeler Foundation.

[a] Mithoefer Center for Rural Surgery, Bassett Healthcare, One Atwell Road, Cooperstown, NY 13326, USA
[b] Department of Surgery, Bassett Healthcare, One Atwell Road, Cooperstown, NY 13326, USA
[c] Department of Surgery, Hospital of Saint Raphael, 1450 Chapel Street, New Haven, CT 06511, USA
* Corresponding author.
E-mail address: steven.heneghan@bassett.org (S.J. Heneghan).

be difficult to provide extensive medical or surgical services on a small, restricted budget. Many rural hospitals, especially those located in small, isolated communities, also struggle to attract and retain qualified staff to deliver medical and surgical care.[4] Patients and their families often prefer to be treated locally, including undergoing surgical procedures, to avoid the added costs and loss of social support that often result when they must travel to a distant regional medical center for surgical care.[5]

Rural hospitals are diverse institutions, and therefore each will have a unique capability to derive economic returns from providing surgical services. The approach to delivering surgical care in rural America varies depending on several factors, including town and service area population, location or proximity to other health care centers, availability and quality of local medical services, community demands and expectations, and the local hospital management's goals.[6] In some cases, a rural hospital may choose to employ a general surgeon directly or grant hospital privileges to a local surgeon who is in solo or group practice. When no surgeon is available locally, the hospital may need to be creative in developing a model to provide surgical care based on its community's unique requirements. This could include any of the following strategies: bringing in general and/or subspecialty surgeons on a regular schedule (or as needed) or using locum tenens surgeons for temporary, ongoing, or on-call coverage.[7] Each of these options has the potential to contribute to a rural hospital's financial health; however, any one option may be more appropriate for a particular hospital, depending on the local situation.

Rural hospitals can derive economic benefits directly and indirectly from the provision of surgical services. A substantial amount of income can be generated directly from surgical procedures that are performed at the local hospital. An examination of billing data conducted in a 1992 Washington State study found that surgical services accounted for 43% of inpatient charges at the state's rural hospitals.[8] In addition, those rural hospitals that had at least 1 general surgeon billed a mean of $1.5 million for surgery. In a rural hospital in southeastern Oregon, over the course of a 2-year period (from 2004 to 2005) the overall hospital revenue increased (by 3.9% and 8.9%, respectively) after the hiring of a full-time general surgeon.[4] According to the hospital auditor, approximately one-third of this increased revenue was derived directly from surgical services. In addition, revenue from associated departments, such as radiology, laboratory, and pharmacy, also increased during this time frame. Providing surgical services can also increase the amount of income that a rural hospital is able to generate by expanding surgery-related services, such as critical care, obstetrics, and trauma. Adding or expanding services that are linked to surgery may ultimately require rural hospitals to hire new staff to increase operating capacity and to attract more patients. This expansion of workforce produces a significant benefit to the local economy.

Rural communities can also derive substantial economic benefits when the local hospital provides surgical services. The health care sector as a whole significantly affects a rural community's economy in various ways. Health care institutions attract external capital as part of the local economic base. They play a role in recruiting associated businesses and employees, and the purchases made by the institution and its employees add dollars to the local economy.[9] According to a 1997 review of the literature on this subject, the health care sector often contributes (through direct and indirect effects) 15% to 20% of a total community's employment and income.[10]

Specifically, hospitals and other health care providers are often one of the largest employers in rural towns along with the government and the education sector. Expanding the number of staff in areas related to surgery, such as nursing and technical operating room positions, can generate added income for the hospital. Rural hospitals and their employees have considerable spending power in rural communities and play a large role in supporting local businesses. A financially strong local hospital that offers a wide range of health care services is also an important yet often overlooked factor in attracting and retaining new businesses, retirees, and workers to a rural community.[9]

In addition to the financial benefits for rural hospitals and communities, there are real costs associated with not having a general surgeon or surgical care available at a rural hospital. Transportation to tertiary care centers for services that could be provided locally if a general surgeon was available is expensive, time consuming, and potentially life-threatening for critically ill patients. In an example from rural southern Arizona, up to 10 emergency patients per month have been flown more than 80 miles to Tucson at a cost of $14,000 per flight since the hospital lost its surgeons.[11] Rural patients and their families who are required to travel for surgical care can incur substantial financial costs and suffer the emotional consequences of being separated from their loved ones during a stressful time.

Without the ability to deliver surgical care, a rural hospital may have to turn away obstetric and emergency cases that rely on surgical backup, potentially leading to greater financial losses. General surgeons often perform most endoscopic procedures, such as colonoscopies, in rural areas where no gastroenterologist is available. If patients are required to travel to regional medical centers for this type of care, bypassing their local rural hospital, they may end up receiving other health care services in the regional centers, thus further draining business. This can lead to the local hospital acquiring a negative reputation as not being able to meet its community's needs, which is a difficult barrier to overcome.[12]

General surgeons and the services they deliver make a significant financial contribution to the health and stability of rural hospitals and communities, whereas the costs incurred when rural residents lack access to local surgical care are great. An ongoing shortage of rural general surgeons, especially in smaller, more isolated regions, makes it difficult for many rural hospitals to provide these services. According to the data published by Thompson and colleagues[13] in 2005, the surgeon to population ratio in small, isolated rural areas was 4.67 per 100,000 compared with 6.53 in urban areas and 7.71 in large rural areas. The results of this study also showed that the average age of surgeons practicing in small rural areas is more than 50 years, suggesting that many will be retiring within the coming decade. One-third to one-half of the surveyed rural hospital administrators stated that they were actively seeking a general surgeon. Their experience shows that recruiting and retaining a qualified general surgeon to practice in a rural hospital is a difficult process, often taking a year or more to accomplish.[1]

Once in rural practice, general surgeons often face significant financial challenges (often including reimbursement at lower rates than their urban counterparts), long work hours, and frequent on-call responsibility that may not be adequately compensated. An option that is becoming more common is for rural hospitals to hire surgeons and pay them a salary to cover many of the expenses that can be difficult to manage in solo rural surgical practice. Hospitals could also benefit from this arrangement by ensuring that they have a stable income from services delivered directly and indirectly as a result of having the surgeon on staff.[14]

Within rural surgery, financial issues have been understudied, resulting in the need for more research on this subject. Few concrete data exist that quantify the economic contribution of a general surgeon to a rural hospital or community. Some available evidence demonstrates the financial value that physicians contribute to local rural hospitals and communities. According to research conducted by the National Center for Rural Health Works at Oklahoma State University, the financial impact made by a typical primary care physician in rural Oklahoma is more than $1 million in direct revenue and more than $720,000 in direct income to a local clinic and hospital.[15] In addition, 12 jobs at the clinic and hospital are created as a result of the business generated through the primary care physician's practice. This type of study must be done to confirm the anecdotal information that shows the significant financial impact that general surgeons have on rural hospitals and communities. Determining which practice models are most financially advantageous for rural surgeons and hospitals is another important area for further study.

Another important question to consider is which surgical procedures general surgeons should be performing in rural hospitals. The typical rural surgeon has a broader case mix than her urban counterparts,[16] and some have argued that with minimal added training, rural general surgeons could perform more than 70% of all inpatient operations at rural hospitals.[17] The capability of a rural hospital to offer the widest possible range of surgical procedures to meet the needs of its residents would seem desirable. From a quality assurance standpoint, however, some might argue that certain lower-volume, more complex procedures should not be done at rural hospitals. A study examining inpatient hospitalizations at rural hospitals in New York State found that there would be minimal financial impact for rural hospitals if most high-risk procedures were referred to regional hospitals.[18]

Answers to these and other related questions should allow rural hospitals and communities to work toward developing strategies for offering surgical care in their areas. Although managing the logistics associated with providing surgical care in the rural setting is complex and may seem daunting in some cases, the financial benefits and equality of patient access resulting from this service are immeasurably valuable to rural patients, hospitals, and communities.

REFERENCES

1. Doty B, Zuckerman R, Finlayson S, et al. General surgery at rural hospitals: a national survey of rural hospital administrators. Surgery 2008;143(5):599–606.
2. Zuckerman R, Doty B, Gold M, et al. General surgery programs in small rural New York State hospitals: a pilot survey of hospital administrators. J Rural Health 2006; 22(4):339–42.
3. Williamson H, Hart G, Piani MJ, et al. Rural hospital inpatient surgical volume: cutting edge service or operating on the margin? J Rural Health 1994;10(1): 16–25.
4. Doty BC, Heneghan S, Zuckerman R. Starting a general surgery program at a small rural critical access hospital: a case study from southeastern Oregon. J Rural Health 2007;23(4):306–13.
5. Finlayson SRG, Birkmeyer JD, Tosteson ANA, et al. Patient preferences for localization of care: implications for regionalization. Med Care 1999;37(2):204–9.
6. Doty B, Zuckerman R, Finlayson S, et al. How does degree of rurality impact the provision of surgical services at rural hospitals? J Rural Health 2008;24(3): 306–10.
7. Doty B, Andres M, Zuckerman R, et al. Use of locum tenens surgeons to provide surgical care in small rural hospitals. World J Surg 2009;33(2):228–32.
8. Williamson H, Hart G, Piani MJ, et al. Market shares for rural inpatient surgical services: where does the buck stop? J Rural Health 1994;10(2):70–9.
9. Scorsone E. Health care services: three critical roles in rural economic development. Economic and policy update. Kentucky Rural Health Works Program. Available at: http://www.ca.uky.edu/krhw/pubs/01oct_roles.html. 2001;01(13). Accessed May 27, 2009.

10. Doeksen GA, Johnson T, Willoughby C. Measuring the economic importance of the health sector on a local economy: a brief literature review and procedures to measure local impacts. Southern Rural Development Center Publication No 202. Available at: http://srdc.msstate.edu/oldsite/publications/202.pdf. 1997. Accessed May 27, 2009.
11. Brown D. Shortage of general surgeons endangers rural Americans. Washington Post 2009. Available at: http://www.washingtonpost.com. Accessed May 17, 2009.
12. Glenn J, Hicks LL, Daugird AJ, et al. Necessary conditions for supporting a general surgeon in rural areas. J Rural Health 1988;4(2):85–100.
13. Thompson M, Lynge DC, Larson EH, et al. Characterizing the general surgery workforce in rural America. Arch Surg 2005;140:75–9.
14. Cofer JB, Burns RP. The developing crisis in the national general surgery workforce. J Am Coll Surg 2008;206(5):790–5.
15. Eilrich FC, Doeksen GA, St. Clair CF. The economic impact of a rural primary care physician and the potential health dollars lost to out-migrating health services. Stillwater (OK): National Center for Rural Health Works. Available at: http://www.ruralhealthworks.org/downloads/Economic/physician_Dollars_Jan_2007.pdf. Accessed May 19, 2009.
16. Ritchie W, Rhodes RS, Biester TW. Workloads and practice patterns of general surgeons in the United States, 1995–1997: a report from the American Board of Surgery. Ann Surg 1999;230(4):533–43.
17. VanBibber M, Zuckerman RS, Finlayson SR. Rural versus urban inpatient case-mix differences in the US. J Am Coll Surg 2006;203(6):812–6.
18. Chappel A, Zuckerman RS, Finlayson SRG. Small rural hospitals and high-risk surgery: how would regionalization affect surgical volume and hospital revenue? J Am Coll Surg 2006;203(5):599–604.

Index

Note: Page numbers of article titles are in **boldface** type.

A

ACS-NSQIP. See *American College of Surgeons National Surgical Quality Improvement Program (ACS-NSQIP).*
American College of Surgeons National Surgical Quality Improvement Program (ACS-NSQIP), 1373, 1379
Australia, rural surgery in, **1325–1333**
    described, 1326–1328
    Mount Gambier, 1330
    Port Augusta, 1329–1330
    Port Lincoln, 1331

B

Bassett healthcare, rural surgery experience, **1321–1323**

C

Community(ies), rural
    financial health of, general surgery as contribution to, **1383–1387**
    interdependence of general surgeons and primary care physicians in, **1293–1302.** See also *General surgeons, primary care physicians and, interdependence of, in rural communities.*
Crossing the Quality Chasm, 1373
Cuyuna Regional Medical Center, in Minnesota, history of, 1352–1354

E

Economy, local, rural surgery's importance to, 1282
Education, for rural surgical practices, **1303–1308.** See also specific areas and *General surgery, in rural areas, education for.*
Endoscopy, training for, at University of Tennessee College of Medicine, 1317

F

Fairness, effects on quality assessment of rural surgery, 1377

G

General surgeons
    in rural areas. See also *Workforce issues, in rural surgery.*
        Australian experience, **1325–1333.** See also *Australia, rural surgery in.*
        broad presence of, 1294
        demographics in, 1280

Surg Clin N Am 89 (2009) 1389–1394
doi:10.1016/S0039-6109(09)00180-7
0039-6109/09/$ – see front matter © 2009 Elsevier Inc. All rights reserved.

surgical.theclinics.com

Moving?

Make sure your subscription moves with you!

To notify us of your new address, find your **Clinics Account Number** (located on your mailing label above your name), and contact customer service at:

Email: journalscustomerservice-usa@elsevier.com

800-654-2452 (subscribers in the U.S. & Canada)
314-447-8871 (subscribers outside of the U.S. & Canada)

Fax number: 314-447-8029

Elsevier Health Sciences Division
Subscription Customer Service
3251 Riverport Lane
Maryland Heights, MO 63043

*To ensure uninterrupted delivery of your subscription, please notify us at least 4 weeks in advance of move.

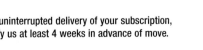
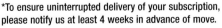